Writing
SOAP Notes
With Patient/Client Management Formats

Writing SOAP Notes

With Patient/Client Management Formats

3rd Edition

GINGE KETTENBACH, PhD, PT
Assistant Professor
Saint Louis University
St. Louis, Missouri

 F.A. DAVIS COMPANY • Philadelphia

Printed in the United States of America

Last digit indicates print number: 10 9 8 7 6 5 4 3 2 1

Acquisitions Editor: Margaret Biblis
Developmental Editor: Michelle L. Clarke
Production Manager: Robert C. Butler
Art and Design Manager: Louis J. Forgione

As new scientific information becomes available through basic and clinical research, recommended treatments and drug therapies undergo changes. The author(s) and publisher have done everything possible to make this book accurate, up to date, and in accord with accepted standards at the time of publication. The author(s), editors, and publisher are not responsible for errors or omissions or for consequences from application of the book, and make no warranty, expressed or implied, in regard to the contents of the book. Any practice described in this book should be applied by the reader in accordance with professional standards of care used in regard to the unique circumstances that may apply in each situation. The reader is advised always to check product information (package inserts) for changes and new information regarding dose and contraindications before administering any drug. Caution is especially urged when using new or infrequently ordered drugs.

Library of Congress Cataloging-in-Publication Data

Kettenbach, Ginge
      Writing SOAP notes / Ginge Kettenbach. — 3rd ed.
          p. cm.
      Title of earlier ed.: Writing S.O.A.P. notes.
      Includes bibliographical references.
      ISBN 0-8036-0836-5
      1. Physical therapy—Problems, exercises, etc. 2. Occupational therapy—Problems, exercises, etc. 3. Medical protocols—Problems, exercises, etc. 4. Note-taking—Problems, exercises, etc. I. Title: Writing S.O.A.P. notes. II. Title.

RM701.6.K48 2003
615.8'2—dc22

Foreword

Almost 10 years have passed since I last worked on the publication of a workbook that built documentation skills. During that time, *The Guide to Physical Therapist Practice* was developed, and evidence-based practice has become part of our vocabulary. Documentation was relatively simple in the early 1990s. One major patient care note format with variations was used by facilities all over the country.

This workbook is an attempt to put the documentation described in *The Guide to Physical Therapist Practice* into real, usable formats. The greatest difficulty is that everyone is not already using some variation of this type of documentation; therefore, I am not describing note formats that are already available. I am instead making an attempt to describe practical note formats, both the SOAP format based on the *Guide to Physical Therapist Practice,* and another format, which I call the Patient/Client Management note format.

Many parts of this workbook will look familiar to those who have used *Writing SOAP Notes* in the past. I certainly used applicable parts of *Writing SOAP Notes* and freely modified other parts to better fit the Patient/Client Management model described in the *Guide to Physical Therapist Practice*. The Patient/Client Management note format is a first try at this format. I imagine in a few years this format will be changed through common usage. I believe this format has merit. Students deserve to know how to write more than one note format.

Books are never written or revised without help and support. I would like to thank the editors at F.A. Davis for their never-ending patience with me in working on this project. My husband Gerry forever encourages me and supports me in every sort of way. Without him, this book would not exist. I would also like to thank my daughters, Kristen and Kathryn, who have grown up watching me write and who now help cover for me when I am too busy to do other things that need to be done in our lives. My final thanks go to my colleagues at Saint Louis University, particularly Theresa Bernsen, who have acted as teachers and sounding boards as I've worked to learn as much as possible about the *Guide to Physical Therapist Practice* and its implications for the real-world practice arena.

Reviewers

Nancy Devine, BS, PT, MS
Instructor
Idaho State University
Pocatello, ID

Terry Chambliss, MhS, PT
Assistant Professor
University of the Sciences in Philadelphia
Philadelphia, PA

Helen Cornely, MS, PT
Associate Professor
Florida International University
Miami, FL

Deborah Edmondson, MS, PT
Assistant Professor/Academic Coordinator
Tennessee State University
Nashville, TN

Cheryl Ford-Smith, MS, PT
Assistant Professor
Medical College of Virginia
Virginia Commonwealth University
Richmond, VA

Brian King, MS, PT
PTA Program Coordinator
Jefferson State Community College
Birmingham, AL

Christine Kowalski, EdD, PTA
PTA Program Director, Chair Allied Health Department
Montana State University—Great Falls
Great Falls, MT

Denise Wise, PT, PhD
Assistant Professor
College of St. Scholastica
Duluth, MN

Contents

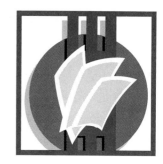

Background Information

D ocumentation is an important part of the care given to every patient. Before a new professional can begin to write notes, some essential information is needed. This section provides the background information that is needed to begin the process of learning to document patient care.

Chapter 1 gives an overview of documentation and the differences and similarities of the two types of patient care notes presented in this text.

Chapter 2 discusses some important basic guidelines that all practitioners should follow when writing in a medical record.

Chapter 3 is a review of medical terminology. Chapter 4 discusses the use of abbreviations and provides an abbreviation list that will be used for all of the worksheets in this text.

The introduction, "How to Use This Book," is essential reading. Completing this book is an exercise that can be very useful, and this introductory material gives guidance on maximizing learning while using this text.

C H A P T E R

1 Introduction to Note Writing

Each day in the clinic, physical and occupational therapists, physical therapist assistants (PTAs), certified occupational therapy assistants (COTAs), and other health care professionals document patient care. One of the methods they use is a form of patient care note called a SOAP Note. Another method is the Patient/Client Management Note.

The SOAP and the Patient/Client Management formats for writing notes are not the only methods used in therapy clinics. However, the SOAP format is commonly used throughout the country, and the Patient/Client Management format is being used as physical therapy practitioners become familiar with the *Guide to Physical Therapist Practice*. It is rare that a health care professional does not encounter one of these two documentation formats, or a variation, during his or her career.

▌What SOAP Means

SOAP is an acronym. Each of the letters in SOAP stands for the name of a section of the patient note.

The patient note is divided as follows:

- **S** stands for *Subjective.*
- **O** stands for *Objective.*
- **A** stands for *Assessment.*
- **P** stands for *Plan.*

In many facilities, a fifth section, the *Problem,* is included before the S portion of the note.

Components of the Patient/Client Management Note

The Patient/Client Management Model described in the *Guide to Physical Therapist Practice* has the following components:

- History
- Systems Review
- Tests and Measures
- Diagnosis
- Prognosis
- Plan of Care

▌The Purposes of Documentation

All health care professionals document their findings for several reasons, including the following:

1. Patient care notes record what the therapist does to manage the individual patient's case. These notes are placed in the patient's medical record. Patient care notes ensure that the rights of the therapist and the patient are protected should any question arise regarding the care provided to the patient. Patient care notes are considered legal documents, as are all parts of the medical record. In the event of litigation, the medical record may be subpoenaed, or the therapist may be called to testify in court or in a deposition on the contents of the medical record.

2. Good documentation is a method of communicating with all other health care professionals, including physicians, other therapists, and therapist assistants. The note communicates the results of the examination, the therapist's evaluation, diagnosis, and prognosis for the patient. It communicates the therapist's (and patient's) expected outcomes and anticipated goals for the patient and the intervention plan, also known as the Plan of Care. The goal of such communication is to provide consistency among the services provided by various health care professionals.

A good patient care note can help a therapist communicate with other therapists or assistants who may provide substitute care for patients during the therapist's absence. The patient care note can be a helpful tool for communication between the therapist and assistant. In a rehabilitation center, school, or other setting using the rehabilitation team approach, the therapist's goals and the patient's level of function can be communicated to other professionals involved in the patient's care. Professionals providing services after the patient is discharged from one therapist's care may find the therapist's notes to be invaluable in planning appropriate follow-up care.

3. Third-party payers, such as Medicare reviewers and representatives from insurance companies, make decisions about reimbursement based on therapy notes. These decisions can be greatly influenced by the quality and completeness of the note.

4. Within the hospital and other types of facilities, patient charts are reviewed. Discharge planning may be based on the notes written by the therapist or assistant. Information that is clearly and correctly documented assists those who are making decisions regarding the patient's disposition and additional care.

5. Writing notes using either the SOAP Note or the Patient/Client Management Note format helps the therapist to organize the thought processes involved in patient care. By thinking in an organized manner, the therapist can better make decisions regarding patient care. Thus, documentation is an excellent method of structuring thinking for clinical decision making.

6. Documentation of patient care can be used for quality assurance and improvement purposes. Standards that indicate and measure quality of care are established. Data can be gathered from the documented records of patient care and evaluated according to predetermined criteria. Results can be used to improve processes or in staff continuing education and professional development activities.

7. Patient care notes can be used in outcomes research. As with quality assurance, certain criteria are initially set for the type of patient to be included and data to be gathered. Data from the notes can be assessed, and conclusions can be drawn about the type of interventions provided for patients with various diagnoses. This type of research is very critical for all health care professionals to ensure high-quality care in a cost-conscious atmosphere. To gather this information, it is vital that health care facilities and groups use a format that is consistent within

their own facilities and with other health care entities. In this way, meaningful and statistically sound data can be compiled.

As a therapist or therapist assistant, it is important to realize that documentation is as integral to the patient care process as the examination, evaluation, or patient intervention. Each day a significant portion of time is spent by therapists and assistants in documenting what is done and why.

Types of Notes

During the course of a patient's care, the patient is initially examined and evaluated, and the therapist generates a diagnosis, prognosis, and Plan of Care. As the Plan of Care is implemented, the patient is re-examined and re-evaluated. Finally, the patient is examined and evaluated on discharge from the therapist's care. Each of these types of examination and evaluation is documented in a type of patient care note. An *initial note* is written after the first patient examination and evaluation and documents the examination, evaluation, diagnosis, prognosis, and Plan of Care. A *progress,* or *interim, note* is written periodically, reporting the results of re-examination and re-evaluation and changes in the prognosis and Plan of Care, as needed. A *discharge note* is written at the time that therapy is discontinued, after a final examination and evaluation are performed. The discharge note addresses the results of the final examination and evaluation, the outcomes and goals achieved, a summary of the interventions received, and the final disposition of the patient.

The Origin of SOAP Notes

The SOAP Note format was introduced by Dr. Lawrence Weed as a part of a system of organizing the medical record, called the problem-oriented medical record (POMR). The POMR has one list of patient problems in the front of the chart, with each health care practitioner writing a separate SOAP Note to address each of the patient's problems. Many facilities never use the POMR; rather, they use some other type of medical record format. Other facilities use an adapted POMR format. In any case, one contribution that clearly came from the POMR was a widespread use of the SOAP Note format.

Professionals in many medical and health fields have adapted the original SOAP format of note writing into a practical tool that is used for documentation. Each field and each facility has its own variation of the SOAP Note. As you enter each clini-

cal facility during your education and later during your professional practice, you will adapt your method of note writing to conform to the variation used by the facility. This workbook will teach you a comprehensive method of writing SOAP Notes that can be adapted to meet the requirements and needs of any facility.

The Patient/Client Management Note

The *Guide to Physical Therapist Practice* was initially published in 1997. After reading the framework for and description of practice published in the *Guide to Physical Therapist Practice,* many physical therapists began to discuss the implications for documentation. Attempts were made by therapists to construct documentation forms and computerized documentation formats that were consistent with this framework of practice.

In the second edition. a Documentation Template was included for initial inpatient and outpatient settings. Some facilities are fully adopting or adapting the Documentation Template for the Patient/Client Management Note. These facilities write patient care notes that use a format that contains all of the elements of the Patient/Client Management Model described in the *Guide to Physical Therapist Practice.* This workbook will teach you to write notes using the Patient/Client Management Note format. This format can be adapted to the needs of any facility.

The Patient/Client Management Process and Documentation Formats

As you approach the process of writing notes, it is necessary to understand the relationship of the SOAP Note and the Patient/Client Management Note to the Patient/Client Management Process. This assists practitioners in determining where information is documented, no matter which note format is used.

The process of clinical decision making used by most therapists includes examining the patient, evaluating the data from the examination, formulating a diagnosis and prognosis, and determining the Plan of Care. Each of these processes is unique, and the results of each process must be documented in the medical record.

Examination

The process of examination includes gathering information from the chart, other caregivers, the patient, the patient's family, caretakers, and friends. It also includes the results of tests and measures performed by the therapist.

In the SOAP Note format, the information gathered in the examination is presented according to the nature of the sources of information. The information gathered from the chart usually is written into an initial section of the note labeled the *Problem*. The information gathered from the patient and the patient's family, caretakers, and friends is usually written into a section labeled the *Subjective (S)* section. Information gathered by the therapist performing tests and measures is usually written into a section labeled the *Objective (O)* section.

In the Patient/Client Management Note format, the information gathered in the examination is divided according to the nature of the data. The information gathered about the patient's history is included in a section labeled *History*. The information gathered from performing a brief examination or screening of the patient's major systems addressed by physical therapy (cardiovascular, integumentary, musculoskeletal, and neuromuscular) is written into a section labeled the *Systems Review*. Information gathered from a brief screening of the patient's communication, affect, cognition, learning style, and education needs is also written into the Systems Review section of the note. Results from specific tests and measures performed by the therapist are documented in a section of the note labeled *Tests and Measures*.

Evaluation

The evaluation process includes synthesis and discussion of clinical findings. In the Patient/Client Management Note format, this information is listed in two sections: the *Diagnosis* and the *Prognosis*. These two sections include a discussion of the issues listed previously, as well as a listing of the *Practice Pattern* from the *Guide to Physical Therapist Practice* (for physical therapists only), the therapy diagnosis and the patient's rehabilitation potential.

In the SOAP Note format, this information appears in the section labeled *Assessment (A)*. The information is written as part of the subsections under "A" labeled *Diagnosis and Prognosis*.

Diagnosis

The *Diagnosis* section of the note includes a discussion of the relationship of the patient's functional deficits to the patient's impairments. If appropriate, a discussion of the relationship of the patient's disability to functional deficits and impairments can be discussed. The patient can be placed in a diagnostic

category as well as in one or more of the practice patterns listed in the *Guide to Physical Therapist Practice*. If more than one practice pattern is applicable, the therapist indicates which practice pattern is primary. A discussion of the relevant functional deficits and impairments, indicating the relevant practice pattern or patterns, may occur in this section. A discussion of other health care professionals to which the therapist has referred the patient or believes the patient should be referred is included in this section. In the SOAP Note, the diagnosis is recorded in the A section of the note in a subsection labeled *Diagnosis*.

Prognosis

The *Prognosis* section of the note in physical therapy includes the predicted level of improvement that the patient will be able to achieve and the predicted amount of time to achieve that level of improvement. This section should also include the therapist's professional opinion of the patient's rehabilitation potential. Future therapy that the therapist believes will be needed after discharge from the therapist's practice setting can be discussed in this section of the note. In the SOAP Note, a discussion of the prognosis and the rationale for the prognosis is recorded in the A section of the note in a subsection labeled *Prognosis*.

Plan of Care

The Plan of Care includes the Expected Outcomes (Long-Term Goals), Anticipated Goals (Short-Term Goals), and Interventions, including an Education Plan for the patient or the patient's caregivers or significant others. The Discharge Plan may also be included in this section of the note. Some facilities may include the Plan of Care with the Prognosis in the note. In both note formats, this information is recorded in a section entitled *Plan of Care (P)*.

Documentation of Health Care Delivery by the Physical Therapist Assistant or Occupational Therapy Assistant

The PTA or COTA reads the initial documentation of the examination, evaluation, diagnosis, prognosis, anticipated outcomes and goals, and intervention plan, and is expected to follow the Plan of Care as outlined by the therapist in the initial patient note. After the patient has been seen by the PTA or COTA for a time (the time varies according to the policies of each facility or health care system and state law), the PTA or COTA must write a progress note documenting any changes in the patient's status that have occurred since the therapist's initial note was written. Also, after discussion with the therapist about the diagnosis and prognosis, expected outcomes, anticipated goals, and interventions, the assistant rewrites or responds to the previously written expected outcomes and documents the revised Plan of Care accordingly. In many facilities, the therapist then cosigns the assistant's notes, indicating agreement with what is documented in the notes. (Once again, this depends on the facility's policies and state law.)

It is extremely important for both therapists and assistants to remember the importance of the role of assistants in documenting patient care. Assistants can develop the skill to participate as fully in documentation of patient care as they do in delivering patient care. With health care delivery continually changing, assisting with documentation is a valuable role for the assistant, and documentation skills are as crucial to the assistant as they are to the therapist. Therefore, PTA and COTA students are encouraged to take full advantage of the skills to be learned from this workbook.

Some of the notes written in the worksheets are examples of initial patient care notes. Although it is acknowledged that the assistant does not write an initial note in the clinic, the same skills used to write initial notes are used to write interim notes. Therefore, assistant students are encouraged to take advantage of the opportunities to write all of the sample notes in all of the worksheets. If it is helpful, think of the examples of initial notes as interim notes during which the therapist and assistant worked together to perform certain patient examinations and discussed the evaluation, diagnosis, prognosis, and revision of the goals and interventions in the Plan of Care. Each facility differs in its use of assistants in both occupational and physical therapy. However, no matter what the specific details of the assistant's role, it is clear that assistants need good documentation skills.

▌ Summary

This workbook will teach you to write two types of documentation, both the Patient/Client Management Note format and the SOAP Note format. Both note formats allow the documentation of patient care and both follow the Patient/Client Management Process described in the *Guide to Physical Therapist Practice*.

The Patient/Client Management Note and SOAP Note formats include the same information. The information is organized differently in each note format, particularly in the way the examination of the patient is documented. The information from the Diagnosis, Prognosis and Plan of Care sections is organized similarly in the two note formats. Appendix B has a chart summarizing the information in the Patient/Client Management Process and the manner in which it is documented in each note format.

Documentation has many purposes, from ensuring quality care to communication to discharge planning. Documentation has become very important in a health care atmosphere that includes litigation, the need of third-party payers to obtain clear and accurate information, and the need for research on the outcomes of the interventions used in rehabilitation. Both methods of writing notes serve as guides to clinical decision making, demonstrating accountability for quality patient care, and documenting patient care.

CHAPTER

2 Writing in a Medical Record

The writing style used in patient care notes at most clinical facilities differs from the style most students are accustomed to using when writing papers, reports, and academic assignments. Writing in patient charts or files requires using medical abbreviations and terminology, and emphasizes brevity. The following guidelines are provided to assist you in becoming accustomed to writing in a medical record.

▌Accuracy

Never record falsely, exaggerate, guess at, or make up data. Patient care notes are parts of a permanent, legal document called the medical record. Incorrect spelling, grammar, and punctuation can be misleading. Objective information, the result of tests and measures that are performed, should be stated in a factual manner.

Keep information objective. Criticisms of other staff members or complaints about working conditions should not be included in the patient care note. The note is about the patient and not about the health care provider.

▌Brevity

Information should be stated concisely. Use short, succinct sentences. Avoid long-winded statements. Also avoid strings of short clauses connected by "and." It is permissible to use sentence fragments or outline form at some facilities. Whatever style is used, it is important to be consistent in style to avoid confusion and to comply with the policies of the facility or practice setting.

Abbreviations can help with brevity. Abbreviations used should be from a list accepted at the facility at which you practice. During your orientation to the facility, you should ask for a copy of that facility's standard list of abbreviations.

 E X A M P L E

Brief
Pt. amb 10 ft. in // bars indep. but required min assist of 1 to turn around in // bars. Sit↔stand from w/c indep. using // bars for support.

Long and Windy
Once the patient wheeled up to the // bars and positioned himself in front of the // bars, he locked his w/c, raised the foot plates, and scooted forward from the seat of the chair. He then gripped the // bars with his hands and on the count of 3 was able to pull himself up to a standing position without any assist. from the therapist. Once standing, he was able to ambulate by positioning his arms forward and then taking steps. He could lead with either right or left foot. Upon turning in the // bars, he was unable to let go with one arm to pivot his body around. Therapist had to give some support until the patient was turned around and both arms were back on the // bars.

Brevity can also be overdone. Enough information must be present to describe pertinent information. Almost every statement in the medical record contains a verb (or some sort of punctuation to replace a verb; see *Punctuation*, following).

▌Clarity

The wording of all patient care notes should be such that the meaning is immediately clear to the reader. Sudden shifts in tense from past to present should be avoided.

Avoid vague terminology.

It is important for handwriting to be legible. The purpose of writing notes is defeated if the notes cannot be easily read.

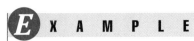

Incorrect
Pt. stated she lived alone. Describes 5 steps s̄ hand railing at entry of her 1-story house. Denied previous use of assist. device.

Correct
States lives alone. Describes 5 steps s̄ hand railing at entry of her 1-story house. Denies previous use of assist. device.

EXAMPLE

Vague
"ROM is ↑" "feeling better" "amb c̄ some assist"

Clear
"Ⓡ shoulder flexion AROM is ↑ to 0–70°"
"Pt. states she knows she is feeling better, indicated by her ability to perform light housekeeping tasks for ≈ 2 hrs ā tiring."
"Pt. amb c̄ walker NWB Ⓛ LE for ≅ 20 ft × 2 c̄ min +1 assist."

Using abbreviations that are standard to the facility is absolutely essential to ensure clarity in note writing. Terminology used within a rehabilitation department, such as *minimal assistance,* or *min assist,* should be well defined and used in a consistent manner by all therapists in the department.

Examples of Errors in Accuracy, Brevity, and Clarity

INCORRECT: Pt. was unable to perform activity due to *muscle absence.* (inaccurate and unclear)
CORRECT: ... due to *muscle paralysis.*

INCORRECT: *Watch for* return of *absent muscles.* (unclear and inaccurate)
CORRECT: *Re-examine* prn for *motor return.*

INCORRECT: Pt. is *sore.* (too brief; unclear)
CORRECT: Pt. is *hypersensitive to touch.*

INCORRECT: Pt. *didn't have any tightness.* (wordy; unclear)
CORRECT: *No ROM limitations* noted.

INCORRECT: Had his Ⓡ leg *cut off because of circulation problems.* (wordy)
CORRECT: Ⓡ transtibial *amputation 2° to PVD.*

INCORRECT: Pt. was unable to wiggle toes *when asked to.* (wordy)
CORRECT: Pt. was unable to wiggle toes *upon request.*

INCORRECT: Examination *was* incomplete *because of* pt. confusion. (wordy and unclear)
CORRECT: Examination incomplete *2° to* pt's inability to follow commands.

Punctuation

Hyphen (-)

Hyphens should be avoided in notes because they can be confused with the minus signs used in muscle grades or negatives (as in SLR:– on Ⓡ). One exception is the common use of a hyphen instead of the word through (as in AROM: 0-48°).

Semicolon (;)

Instead of overusing "states" in the subjective part of the note, a semicolon can be used to connect two related statements.

EXAMPLE

Wordy
"States position of comfort for sleep is on Ⓡ side. States pain does not awaken Pt. at night."

Brief
"States position of comfort for sleep is on Ⓡ side; pain does not awaken Pt. at night."

Colon (:)

A colon can be used instead of "is."

EXAMPLE

Instead of "AROM Ⓡ shoulder flexion is 0–90°," you could say "AROM Ⓡ shoulder flexion: 0–90°."

Correcting Errors

Correction fluid or tape should *not* be used on a medical record. Trying to destroy or attempting to obliterate information makes it look as if the health professional is trying to "cover up" malpractice. The proper method of correcting a charting mistake is to put a line through the error, write the date and initial it above the error.

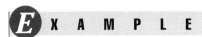

Correct
vkk 2/28/03
~~some~~ min +1 assist.

Signing Your Notes

You should sign every entry that you make into the medical record. All notes should be signed with your legal signature (your last name and legal first name or initials). No nicknames should be used. Initials should follow your name indicating your status as a therapist or therapist assistant.

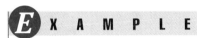

Sue Brown, PT or James Smith, PTA
Maryann Jones, OTR or B. J. McDonald, COTA

In some facilities, there is a custom of using additional initials prior to PT or PTA (L, P, or R). The American Physical Therapy Association advocates the use of PT or PTA only. The American Occupational Association advocates the use of OTR or COTA. In some clinics, students sign their notes SPT or SPTA, OTS or OTAS. In others, students are required to sign their name only. In either case, the signature of a student should always be followed by a slash and then the signature of the supervising therapist.

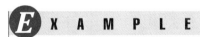

Gene White, SPT/Sue Brown, PT
Peter Maxwell, OTS/Maryann Jones, OTR

Referring to Yourself

Notes discuss the patient and not the therapist.

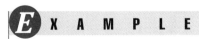

Incorrect
I helped this patient transfer c̄ min assist. from his w/c to the plinth.

Correct
Pt. transferred c̄ min assist. w/c↔plinth.

If for some reason a therapist must make reference to himself or herself, most facilities prefer that the reference be made in the third person as *therapist, physical therapist,* or *occupational therapist.*

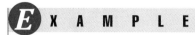

Pt. states therapist should be putting his shoes on for him like his family does at home.

Blank or Empty Lines

Empty lines should not be left between one entry and another, nor should empty lines be left within a single entry. Empty lines are areas in which another person could falsify information already charted. Adding even one word, such as *not,* to a note can completely change the meaning of the note's content.

Writing Orders in a Chart

When a physician gives an order to a therapist, the therapist is the professional responsible for writing it in the chart. In writing an order in the chart, the following format is standard in most facilities:

date/time/order
v.o. physician's name/therapist's signature, OTR (or PT)

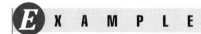

12-24-2001/10:50/Pt. may be FWB in PT
v.o. Dr. Ache/Sue Brown, PT

Once the order is written by the therapist in the chart, the physician cosigns the order the next time he or she sees the chart or as soon as possible thereafter.

Summary

Writing in a medical record should be brief, accurate, and clear. Errors should be corrected, *not* erased or covered with correction fluid. You should use your legal signature as you would on any legal document. If you follow these guidelines and apply them throughout the exercises in this book, with time you will develop a good medical writing style that you will use daily in clinical practice.

3 Medical Terminology

Before any health care professional can begin reading or writing medical documentation in an acceptable manner, she or he must be familiar with the terminology commonly used in medical writing. Most of the terms have Greek- or Latin-based prefixes, suffixes, or roots. It is often easy to ascertain the meaning of a particular term if the more commonly used prefixes, suffixes, and roots are known.

Learning medical terminology and its prefixes, suffixes, and roots is outside the scope of this workbook. Some basic knowledge of medical terminology is assumed.

The following worksheets should serve as a review of medical terminology. The terms used in these worksheets are encountered frequently by therapists and assistants. If you are unfamiliar with the terms and definitions used in these worksheets, it is suggested that you review medical terminology before continuing in this workbook. The list of references in Appendix F of this book should prove helpful to you in reviewing medical terminology, if needed.

term = prefix + *root* or	*Example:* Sclero*derma*
term = *root* + suffix or	*Example:* Osteoporosis
term = prefix + *root* + suffix	*Example:* Syn*dactyl*ism

Medical Terminology:
WORKSHEET 1

PART I. Write the appropriate term for the definition.

1. Tumor of the bone _____

2. Abnormally low blood sugar _____

3. Beneath the skin _____

4. Above the symphysis pubis _____

5. Pertaining to the back of the body _____

6. Toward the head _____

7. Abnormal redness of the skin _____

8. Between the ribs _____

9. Front of the body _____ or

_____

10. Conducting toward a structure _____

PART II. Write the appropriate definition for the term listed.

1. Symphysis pubis

_____

_____

2. Cardiomegaly

_____

_____

3. Meniscectomy

_____

_____

4. Chondroma

_____

_____

5. Arthrodesis

_____

_____

6. Craniotomy

_____

_____

7. Neurology

_____

_____

8. Anesthesia

_____

_____

9. Phlebitis

_____

_____

10. Hypertension

_____

_____

Answers to "Medical Terminology: Worksheet 1" are provided in Appendix A.

Medical Terminology:
WORKSHEET 2

2

PART I. Write the appropriate term for the definition.

1. Joint inflammation
    _____

2. Inspection of joint with a scope
    _____

3. Disease of a muscle
    _____

4. Difficult or bad breathing
    _____

5. Lack of coordination
    _____

6. Softening of cartilage
    _____

7. Inflammation of the brain
    _____

8. Tumor of the meninges
    _____

9. Paralysis of one half of the body
    _____

10. Beneath the clavicle
    _____

PART II. Write the appropriate definition for the term listed.

1. Analgesia:
_____
_____

2. Bilateral:
_____
_____

3. Contralateral:
_____
_____

4. Aphasia:
_____
_____

5. Tendinitis:
_____
_____

6. Bradykinesia:
_____
_____

7. Dysphagia:

_____

_____

8. Arthralgia:

_____

_____

9. Cerebromalacia:

_____

_____

10. Costochondral:

_____

_____

Answers to "Medical Terminology: Worksheet 2" are provided in Appendix A.

CHAPTER

4 Using Abbreviations

Abbreviations are used to save time and space while writing notes. To ensure that everyone involved in the patient's care can understand what has been written in the chart by others, most medical facilities have a list of approved abbreviations, and these are the only abbreviations that should be used in that particular facility. A committee at each facility approves this list. The list of acceptable abbreviations varies from one facility to the next.

The list of abbreviations that follows will be used

as the approved list for all of the worksheets in this book. Any abbreviations not on this list are considered unacceptable for these worksheets. When you begin your career, please remember that the list of acceptable abbreviations for your clinical facility must be used. During orientation to any clinical facility in which you practice, you should ask about the location of the approved abbreviations list and become particularly familiar with the abbreviations used frequently by the facility. For further reference on abbreviations, see Appendix E.

Approved Abbreviations and Symbols for Hospital XYZ

A:	assessment
ABI	acquired brain injury
afib	atrial fibrillation
A-line	arterial line
A-V	arteriovenous
AAA	abdominal aortic aneurysm
AAROM	active assistive range of motion
Abd or abd	abduction
ABG	arterial blood gases
ac	before meals
AC joint	acromioclavicular joint
ACL	anterior cruciate ligament
ACTH	adrenocorticotrophic hormone
Add or add	adduction
ADL	activities of daily living
ad lib	at discretion
adm	admission, admitted
AE	above elbow
AFO	ankle foot orthosis
AIDS	acquired immune deficiency syndrome
AIIS	anterior inferior iliac spine
AJ	ankle jerk
AK	above knee

ALS	amyotrophic lateral sclerosis
a.m.	morning
AMA	against medical advice
amb	ambulation, ambulating, ambulated, ambulate, ambulates
ANS	autonomic nervous system
ant	anterior
AP	anterior-posterior
ARDS	adult respiratory distress syndrome
ARF	acute renal failure
AROM	active range of motion
ASA	aspirin
ASAP or asap	as soon as possible
ASCVD	arteriosclerotic cardiovascular disease
ASHD	arteriosclerotic heart disease
ASIS	anterior superior iliac spine
assist.	assistance, assistive
AVM	arteriovenous malformation

B/S	bedside
BBB	bundle branch block
BE	below elbow
BID or bid	twice a day
bilat. or Ⓑ	bilateral, bilaterally
BK	below knee
BM	bowel movement
BOS	base of support
BP	blood pressure
bpm	beats per minute
BR	bedrest
BRP	bathroom privileges
BS	breath sounds or bowel sounds
BUN	blood urea nitrogen (blood test)

C	centigrade
C&S	culture and sensitivity
c/o	complains of
CA	cancer, carcinoma
CABG	coronary artery bypass graft
CAD	coronary artery disease
cal	calories
CAT	computerized axial tomography
CBC	complete blood cell (count)
CC, C/C	chief complaint
cc	cubic centimeter
CF	cystic fibrosis
CHF	congestive heart failure
cm	centimeter
CMV	cytomegalovirus
CNS	central nervous system
CO	cardiac output
CO_2	carbon dioxide
cont.	continue
COPD	chronic obstructive pulmonary disease

COTA	certified occupational therapy assistant
CP	cerebral palsy
CPAP	continuous positive airway pressure
CPR	cardiopulmonary resuscitation
CRF	chronic renal failure
CSF	cerebral spinal fluid
CV	cardiovascular
CWI	crutch walking instructions
CXR	chest x-ray
Cysto	cystoscopic examination
D/C	discontinued or discharged
dept.	department
DIP	distal interphalangeal (joint)
DJD	degenerative joint disease
DM	diabetes mellitus
DNR	do not resuscitate
DO	doctor of osteopathy
DOB	date of birth
DOE	dyspnea on exertion
DTR	deep tendon reflex
DVT	deep vein thrombosis
Dx	diagnosis
ECF	extended care facility
ECG, EKG	electrocardiogram
ED	emergency department
EEG	electroencephalogram
EENT	ear, eyes, nose, throat
EMG	electromyogram, electromyography
E.R.	emergency room
eval.	evaluation
ext.	extension
FBS	fasting blood sugar
FEV	forced expiratory volume
FH	family history
flex	flexion
FRC	functional residual capacity
ft.	foot, feet (the measurement, not the body part)
FUO	fever, unknown origin
FVC	forced vital capacity
FWB	full weight bearing
fx	fracture
GB	gallbladder
GI	gastrointestinal
g	gram
GSW	gunshot wound
GYN	gynecology
h, hr.	hour

H&H, H/H	hematocrit and hemoglobin
H&P	history and physical
h/o	history of
HA, H/A	headache
Hb, Hgb	hemoglobin
Hct	hematocrit
HCVD	hypertensive cardiovascular disease
HEENT	head, ear, eyes, nose, throat
HEP	home exercise program
HIV	human immunodeficiency virus
HNP	herniated nucleus pulposus
HOB	head of bed
HR	heart rate
hr.	hour
hs	at bedtime
ht.	height
Ht	hematocrit
Htn or HTN	hypertension
Hx	history

I&O	intake and output
IADL	instrumental activities of daily living
ICU	intensive care unit
IDDM	insulin dependent diabetes mellitus
IM	intramuscular
imp.	impression
in.	inches
indep	independent
IMV	intermittent mandatory ventilation
inf	inferior
IRDS	infant respiratory distress syndrome
IS	incentive spirometry
IV	intravenous

KAFO	knee ankle foot orthosis
kcal	kilocalories
kg	kilogram
KJ	knee jerk
KUB	kidney, ureter, bladder

L or l.	liter
Ⓛ	left
lat	lateral
lb.	pound
LBBB	left bundle branch block
LBP	low back pain
LE	lower extremity
LOC	loss of consciousness, level of consciousness
LMN	lower motor neuron
LOS	length of stay
LP	lumbar puncture

m	meter
MAP	mean arterial pressure
max	maximal
MD	medical doctor; doctor of medicine
MED	minimal erythemal dose
Meds.	medications
mg	milligram
MI	myocardial infarction
min	minimal
min.	minute
ml	milliliter
mm	millimeter
MMT	manual muscle test
mo.	month
mod	moderate
MP, MEP	metacarpophalangeal
MRSA	methicillin resistant staphylococcus aureus
MS	multiple sclerosis
MVA	motor vehicle accident

NDT	neurodevelopmental treatment
neg.	negative
NG or ng	nasogastric
N.H.	nursing home
NIDDM	non-insulin–dependent diabetes mellitus
nn	nerve
noc	night, at night
NPO or npo	nothing by mouth
NSR	normal sinus rhythm
NWB	non-weight bearing

O:	objective
OA	osteoarthritis
OB	obstetrics
OBS	organic brain syndrome
od	once daily
OOB	out of bed
O.P.	outpatient
O.R.	operating room
ORIF	open reduction, internal fixation
OT	occupational therapy, occupational thrapist
OTR	occupational therapist (used to follow official signature of the occupational therapist)
oz.	ounce

P	poor
P:	plan (intervention plan)
P.A.	physician's assistant
PA	posterior/anterior
para	paraplegia
pc	after meals
PCL	posterior cruciate ligament

PE	pulmonary embolus
PEEP	positive end expiratory pressure
per	by/through
p.o.	by mouth
PERRLA	pupils equal, round, reactive to light, and accommodation
P.H.	past history
p.m.	afternoon
PMH	past medical history
PNF	proprioceptive neuromuscular facilitation
PNI	peripheral nerve injury
POMR	problem-oriented medical record
pos.	positive
poss	possible
post	posterior
post-op	after surgery (operation)
PRE	progressive resistive exercise
pre-op	before surgery (operation)
prn	whenever necessary, as often as necessary
PROM	passive range of motion
PSIS	posterior superior iliac spine
PT	physical therapy, physical therapist (used after therapist's signature)
PT/PTT	prothrombin time/partial thromboplastin time
Pt., pt.	patient
PTA	physical therapist assistant
PTA	prior to admission
PTB	patellar tendon bearing
PVD	peripheral vascular disease
PWB	partial weight bearing

q	every
qd	every day
qh	every hour
qid	four times a day
qn	every night
qt.	quart

Ⓡ	right
RA	rheumatoid arthritis
RBBB	right bundle branch block
RBC	red blood cell (count)
R.D.	registered dietician
re:	regarding
rehab	rehabilitation
reps	repetitions
resp	respiratory, respiration
RN	registered nurse
R/O or r/o	rule out
ROM	range of motion
ROS	review of systems
RR	respiratory rate
RROM	resistive range of motion
R.T.	respiratory therapist, respiratory therapy
Rx	intervention plan, prescription, therapy

SACH	solid ankle cushion heel
SCI	spinal cord injury
SC joint	sternoclavicular joint
sec.	seconds
SED	suberythemal dose
sig	directions for use, give as follows, let it be labeled
SI(J)	sacroiliac (joint)
SLE	systemic lupus erythematosus
SLP	speech-language pathologist
SLR	straight leg raise
SNF	skilled nursing facility
SOAP	subjective, objective, assessment, plan
SOB	shortness of breath
S/P	status post (e.g., "S/P hip fx" means "Pt. fx her hip in the recent past.")
spec	specimen
stat.	immediately, at once
sup	superior
Sx	symptoms
tab	tablet
TB	tuberculosis
TBI	traumatic brain injury
tbsp.	tablespoon
TENS, TNS	transcutaneous electrical nerve stimulator or transcutaneous electrical nerve stimulation
THA	total hip arthroplasty
ther ex	therapeutic exercise
TIA	transient ischemic attack
tid	three times daily
TKA	total knee arthroplasty
TM(J)	temporomandibular (joint)
TNR	tonic neck reflex (also ATNR, STNR)
t.o.	telephone order
TPR	temperature, pulse, and respiration
tsp.	teaspoon
TUR	transurethral resection
Tx	traction
TV	tidal volume
UA	urine analysis
UE	upper extremity
UMN	upper motor neuron
URI	upper respiratory infection
US	ultrasound
UTI	urinary tract infection
UV	ultraviolet
VC	vital capacity
VD	venereal disease
v.o. or VO	verbal orders (e.g., v.o. Dr. Smith/assistant's signature)
vol.	volume
v.s.	vital signs

w/c	wheelchair
W/cm²	watts per square centimeter
WBC	white blood cell (count)
wk.	week
WNL	within normal limits
wt.	weight
x	number of times performed (e.g., x2 is twice; x3 is 3 times)
y/o or y.o.	years old
yd.	yard
yr.	year
+1, +2	assistance (assistance of 1 person given; also written "assistance of 1." Examples: amb … c̄ min + 1 assist., or amb … c̄ +1 min assist., or amb … c̄ min assist. of 1)
♂	male
♀	female
↓	down, downward, decrease, diminished
↑	up, upward, increase, augmented
//	parallel or parallel bars (also written "// bars")
c̄	with
s̄	without
p̄	after
ā	before
~ or ≈	approximately
@	at (this symbol is not exclusively used for *at*)
Δ	change
>	greater than
<	less than
=	equal
+ or (+)	plus, positive (positive also abbreviated "pos.")
− or (−)	minus, negative (negative also abbreviated "neg.")
#	number (#1 = number 1), pounds (5# wt. = 5 pound weight; *pound* also abbreviated "lbs.")
/	per
%	percent
+, &, et.	and
↔, ⇌, or ⇄	to and from
→	to progressing toward, approaching
1°	primary
2°	secondary, secondary to

▌Using Abbreviations: Examples

The following are examples of the use of abbreviations in medical records.

1. In the physician's notes, you may find the following: Pt. has hx of Htn, ASHD, CHF, MI in 2000, TIA in 2001.

   Translation: The patient has a history of hypertension, arteriosclerotic heart disease, congestive heart failure, myocardial infarction in 2000, transient ischemic attack in 2001.

2. Orders written in the chart:
   Up ad lib
   ASA q 4h
   BRP prn
   NPO p̄ midnight
   v.o. Dr. Smith/Janice Jones, OTR

   Translation:
   Up at discretion (patient's discretion)
   Aspirin every 4 hours
   Bathroom privileges when necessary
   Nothing by mouth after midnight
   Verbal order given by Dr. Smith to Janice Jones, occupational therapist

3. In PT note: Rx: AROM Ⓡ ankle bid

   Translation: Treatment intervention: Active range of motion right ankle two times per day.

4. In chart in doctor's initial note: imp: COPD; R/O lung CA

   Translation: Impression: Chronic obstructive pulmonary disease; rule out lung cancer.

5. Physician's orders: Record I&O; all meds per IV; NPO; transfer pt. to ICU

   Translation: Record intake and output.
   All medications through intravenous tube.
   Nothing by mouth.
   Transfer patient to the intensive care unit.

You will be expected to be able to both interpret and use abbreviations in the medical record. You will encounter most of the abbreviations listed in this chapter when you practice in the clinic. Any time you write a note, you will be expected to use abbreviations properly.

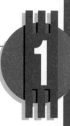

Translate each phrase or sentence written with abbreviations into a full English phrase or sentence. Translate each sentence or phrase written in English into a sentence or phrase written with abbreviations.

1. <u>Physician's orders</u>:

   to PT per w/c turn Pt. qh

   Translation:
   _____
   _____
   _____

2. <u>In chart</u>:

   Dx: RA; R/O SLE

   Translation:
   _____
   _____

3. <u>In PT note</u>:

   Intervention plan: once per day, activities of daily living training, ultrasound to 1.0 to 1.5 watts per centimeter squared to anterior superior aspect of right knee for 5 minutes.

   Translation:
   _____
   _____
   _____
   _____

4. <u>In OT or PT note</u>:

   c/o SOB p̄ bilat. UE PNF exercises.

   Translation:
   _____
   _____
   _____
   _____
   _____

5. <u>In chart</u>:

   Dx: MS; R/O OBS.

   Translation:
   _____
   _____
   _____

6. <u>In PT note</u>:

   The patient has a below-the-knee amputation. Has used a patellar tendon bearing prosthesis with a solid ankle cushion heel foot for the past 20 years.

   Translation:
   _____
   _____
   _____

7. <u>In OT note</u>:

   The patient's heart rate increased 20 beats per minute after only 2 minutes of self-care activities of daily living.

   Translation:
   _____
   _____
   _____

8. <u>In PT note</u>:

   The patient ambulated in the parallel bars, full weight bearing left lower extremity, for approximately 20 feet twice with minimal assistance of one person.

   <u>Translation</u>:

   _____

   _____

   _____

9. <u>In OT or PT note</u>:

   Upper extremity strength is 5/5 throughout bilaterally.

   <u>Translation</u>:

   _____

   _____

10. <u>In PT or OT note</u>:

    Anticipated Goal: decrease dependence in transfers wheelchair to bed to moderate assistance within 1 week.

    <u>Translation</u>:

    _____

    _____

Answers to "Using Abbreviations: Worksheet 1" are included in Appendix A.

1. Pt. c/o Ⓡ hip pain $\bar{p}$ amb ≈ 300 ft. x 1 $\bar{c}$ a walker FWB Ⓡ LE.

Translation:

_____

_____

_____

_____

2. <u>You must write in the chart:</u> The patient may be 50 percent partial weight-bearing left lower extremity per verbal order of Dr. Smith.

Translation:

_____

_____

_____

3. <u>Order written in chart:</u> D/C US in area of Ⓡ SI joint.

Translation:

_____

_____

_____

4. <u>Medical Dx:</u> Fx Ⓛ clavicle & subluxation Ⓛ SC joint.

Translation:

_____

_____

_____

_____

5. <u>In physician's note:</u> FBS upon adm was over 300.

Translation:

_____

_____

_____

6. The medical diagnosis is left chronic renal failure.

Translation:

_____

7. The muscle function test reveals strength 4/5 throughout the upper extremities bilaterally.

Translation:

_____

_____

_____

_____

8. X-ray examination reveals fracture of the left third metacarpal immediately proximal to the metacarpophalangeal joint.

Translation:

_____

_____

_____

_____

9. <u>Order for you to write in the chart</u>: To occupational therapy for activities of daily living per verbal order of Dr. Jones.

Translation:

_____

_____

10. <u>In the physician's note</u>: Imp: peripheral neuropathy; R/O CNS dysfunction.

Translation:

_____

_____

_____

_____

Answers to "Using Abbreviations: Worksheet 2" are provided in Appendix A.

Documenting the Examination

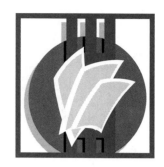

When a therapist sees a patient for the first time, the therapist performs an examination. This examination leads to the therapist's evaluation and determination of the diagnosis, prognosis, and plan of care for the patient. Therefore, documenting the results of the examination performed by the therapist is a very important part of documenting patient care.

As mentioned in chapter 1, the examination is documented differently in the SOAP and Patient/Client Management note formats. The SOAP note format organizes the information according to the source of the information. The Patient/Client Management note format organizes the information by the patient/client management processes that occur in patient care.

This section first presents the three subsections of the Examination part of the Patient/Client Management note (Chapters 5–7). Then it presents the Problem, S, and O sections of the SOAP note (Chapters 6–8). Worksheets follow the chapters to allow you to practice and gain confidence in documenting these sections of the two note formats.

CHAPTER

5 The Patient/Client Management Format: History

The first part of the Patient/Client Management note is the Examination. The Examination section includes three subsections. The first subsection is entitled *History*. The second subsection is entitled *Systems Review*. The third subsection is entitled *Tests and Measures*. Information belongs under History if it includes the following:

● Demographic information about the patient known as **identifying information:** This information includes the patient's name, address, admission date, date of birth, sex, dominant hand, race, ethnicity, language, education level, advance directive preferences, referral source, and reasons for referral to therapy.

● The patient's **current conditions/chief complaints:** This includes the onset date of the problem, any incident that caused or contributed to the onset of the problem, prior history of similar problems, how the patient is caring for the problem, what makes the problem better and worse, patient goals for therapy, and any other practitioner the patient is seeing for the problem.

● The patient's **social history:** The social history

includes cultural and religious beliefs that might affect care, the person(s) with whom the patient lived prior to admission and will live after discharge, available social and physical supports available to the patient now and that will be available after discharge, and the availability of a caregiver.

● The patient's **employment status:** This includes whether the patient works full time or part time, inside or outside of the home, is retired, or is a student.

● A description of the patient's **living environment:** This includes the devices and equipment the patient uses, the type of residence in which the patient lives, information about the environment such as stairs or ramps available, and past use of community services. Community services can include day services or programs, home health services, homemaking services, hospice, Meals on Wheels, mental health services, respiratory therapy, or one of the rehabilitation therapies (physical therapy, occupational therapy, speech language pathology).

● Information about the patient's **general health status:** This includes the patient's rating of his or her health and whether the patient has experienced any major life changes during the preceding year.

● Information about the patient's past and current **social/health habits:** This includes alcohol and tobacco use and exercise habits.

● Information about the patient's **family health history:** This is a general screening for a family history of heart disease, hypertension, stroke, diabetes, cancer, psychologic conditions, arthritis, osteoporosis, and other conditions.

● Information about the **patient's medical/surgical history.**

● Information about the **functional status/activity level** of the patient: This includes information on everything from bed mobility, transfers, gait, self-care, home management, and community and work activities that apply to the patient's current situation or condition.

● A current list of all of the **medications** the patient takes.

● The **growth and development** of the patient: This includes the developmental history and is most applicable to pediatric patients.

● **Other clinical tests** that the patient has experienced: This includes laboratory tests or radiologic tests, and the dates and the findings of those tests.

Although the therapist makes every attempt at performing a complete examination of the patient, not every category may be used with every patient. For example, the developmental category may not be applicable to an older adult with degenerative joint disease.

▌Use of the Term *Patient*

Much of the information in the History section of the note is obtained from the patient or the patient's family or friends. Therefore, many statements in the History part of the note may refer to the patient. It is unnecessary to refer to the source of information unless information from two sources conflicts despite the therapist's attempts to clarify discrepancies, or unless the information is clearly the patient's opinion or belief and not factual or documented medically.

 X A M P L E

Functional Status/Activity Level: Pt. states she performs all transfers indep. & safely. Pt's daughter states Pt. lives in assisted living situation because Pt. falls frequently & needs help c̄ transfers @ times.

Current Condition: Pt. states she believes the pain in her foot is caused by her back.

▌Abbreviations and Medical Terminology

Appropriate abbreviations and use of medical terminology are expected. Correct spelling is necessary for the therapist to be represented appropriately as a professional. The most concise (yet clear) wording should be used. Full sentences are not necessary if the idea is complete (this varies from facility to facility). If the information does not conflict, it is not necessary to identify the source of the information.

 X A M P L E

Wordy: The patient's daughter stated that she talked with her mother and that her mother will go to the daughter's home upon discharge from the hospital.

More Concise: Pt. will go to daughter's home p̄ D/C.

Organization

Other health care professionals reading your note need to be able to find the information in your note. Therefore, the use of headings or subcategories is important. The headings used are the same as the types of information included in the History subsection of the note. To which of the two following examples would you rather refer if you were looking for particular information?

> **E X A M P L E**
>
> 1. Works full time inside of the home doing data entry. Lives in a house c̄ 4 stairs to enter. Pt. rates general health as fair. No railings on the stairs. Denies major life changes during past yr. Sidewalk between garage & house is uneven surface. Lives alone.
> 2. <u>Social History:</u> Lives alone. <u>Employment:</u> Works full time inside of home doing data entry. <u>Living Environment:</u> Lives in a house c̄ 4 stairs s̄ railings to enter. Sidewalk between garage & house is uneven surface. <u>General Health Status:</u> Rates general health as fair. Denies major life changes during past yr.

In the first example, getting a picture of the patient's home status, work status, and health status is difficult. The second example is much easier to read and understand.

Every initial note should include applicable information on the patient's *identifying (or demographic) information, current conditions and chief complaints, social history, employment or work status, living environment, general health status, social and health habits, family health history, patient medical/surgical history, functional status and activity level, medications, and other clinical tests. Growth and development* is an optional subcategory. The information under each subcategory should be as brief and concise as possible. The purpose of the information is not to add length to the note, but to provide necessary documentation of the patient's history.

Progress, or Interim, Notes

Progress note formats for the Patient/Client Management format vary. In some facilities, the History subsection of a progress note is written using only the categories that need to be updated.

Other facilities use the SOAP note format to document patient progress. Each individual health care facility has policies regarding how to document updates to the information included in the History part of the note.

Discharge Summaries

In some health care facilities, the History section of the Discharge Summary is used as a summary of the patient's history, including progress or changes made in certain areas during the course of care. Some subsections under History remain unchanged (unless the information was corrected) from the initial note. Other subsections summarize the changes made while the patient received therapy.

> **E X A M P L E**
>
> From a single subheading of the History section of the note:
>
> *Current Conditions/Chief Complaint:* Pt. initially c/o low back pain of an intensity of 8 on a 0–10 scale. Pt. was pain free upon D/C. Pt. stated she learned she had to do her exercises daily to remain pain free.

Other health care facilities omit the History section from the Discharge Summary.

Summary

The History is the first section of the Examination part of the Patient/Client Management note. It should include subheadings with information regarding the patient's identifying information (demographics), current conditions and chief complaints, social history, employment or work situation, living environment, general health status, social and health habits, family history, patient or client medical/surgical history, functional status and activity level, medications, and other clinical tests. The history should be written in a concise method, using appropriate abbreviations and spelling.

The worksheets that follow will give you practice writing the History portion of the Examination Section of a Patient/Client Management Note. After reviewing the material in this chapter, completing the following worksheets, and using the answer sheets to correct the worksheets, you will be able to write the History subsection of a Patient/Client Management Note.

Writing History:
Worksheet 1

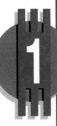

PART I. Mark the statements that should be placed in the *History* category by placing an *H* on the line before the statement.

1. _____ Pt. best learns through reading and demonstration.

2. _____ Communication abilities: WNL.

3. _____ Pt. is a 31 y.o. white male referred by Dr. Smith c̄ a medical dx of S/P fx Ⓡ femur 6 wks. ago.

4. _____ Integumentary system: skin color and integrity WNL.

5. _____ Prior Rx: PT in ED for training in gait c̄ crutches.

6. _____ Lives c̄ his wife & 2 children.

7. _____ Pt. is indep. in all transfer, ADL, & IADL activities.

8. _____ Balance is not impaired.

9. _____ Oriented × 3.

10. _____ Pt. works full time as a postal worker & has been on leave of absence for past 6 wks.

11. _____ Education needs: exercise program & recovery process from fx.

12. _____ Pt referred for gait training s̄ assistive device.

13. _____ Denies major life changes during the past year.

14. _____ Rates general health as excellent.

15. _____ Gross locomotion NWB c̄ crutches is not impaired; has been NWB Ⓡ LE for 6 wks.

PART II. Below you will find the headings discussed for the *History* subsection of the note. Each is followed by five blanks (more than are needed for the exercise). Below these headings are twenty statements to be included in the note. Write the number of each in the blank following its appropriate heading. The statements you list following each heading should be in the order in which they would logically appear in a note (for instance, 1-5-3 might make more sense than if you were to order them 3-1-5). You may wish to write the note out on a separate piece of paper to assist yourself with this task.

A. <u>Demographics:</u> ____, ____ , ____ , ____ , ____

B. <u>Current Condition(s)/Chief Complaint(s):</u> ____, ____ , ____ , ____ , ____

C. <u>Social Hx:</u> ____, ____ , ____ , ____ , ____

D. <u>Employment/Work:</u> ____, ____ , ____ , ____ , ____

E. <u>Living Environment:</u> ____, ____ , ____ , ____ , ____

F. <u>General Health Status:</u> ____, ____ , ____ , ____ , ____

G. <u>Social/Health Habits:</u> ____, ____ , ____ , ____ , ____

H. Family Hx: ____ , ____ , ____ , ____ , ____

I. Medical/Surgical Hx: ____ , ____ , ____ , ____ , ____

J. Functional Status/Activity Level: ____ , ____ , ____ , ____ , ____

K. Medications: ____ , ____ , ____ , ____ , ____

L. Other Clinical Tests: ____ , ____ , ____ , ____ , ____

1. Perceives general health as good.
2. Pt. lap swims 1.5 hrs. 5x/wk.
3. c/o pain c̄ wt. bearing Ⓡ ankle.
4. X-rays were neg.
5. Referred by Dr. Jones.
6. Unable to play bass in church (stands for this activity).
7. Home has 1 step to enter & is on 1 level.
8. Walking at school is painful.
9. Cannot stand during bass lessons.
10. 13 y.o.
11. Wears an ankle wrap when swimming.
12. Medical dx of S/P sprain Ⓡ ankle 4 wks.
13. Rates pain as 4 on a 0–10 scale (0 = no pain).
14. female
15. Has not received any Rx of this Ⓡ ankle sprain other than splinting.
16. Hx of 3 previous Ⓡ ankle sprains & 2 previous Ⓡ wrist sprains.
17. Caucasian
18. Pain is limiting Pt's recreational activities in middle school; unable to participate in after-school art activities due to pain level at end of day.
19. Pt. goal: to amb. pain free s̄ splint Ⓡ LE.
20. Lives c̄ parents.
21. Pt. does not smoke or drink.
22. Pt is Ⓡ handed.
23. Attends middle school.
24. School has 2 levels c̄ 2 flights of 10 steps between levels.
25. Currently takes 400 mg. of ibuprofen TID for pain.
26. Is on swim team at local YMCA.
27. Pt. fell on a step at home & "severely" twisted Ⓡ ankle medially on [date].
28. Plays bass in orchestra at school.
29. Grandparents had HCVD, father has Htn, sister dx c̄ connective tissue disease; family could not remember name of connective tissue disease.
30. Currently wearing splint on Ⓡ ankle.

PART III. Rewrite the following History statements in a more clear, concise, and professional manner. Also, list the heading under which the statement should be placed.

1. The patient is an 83-year-old woman who is African-American and who is right-handed.

    a. Heading: _____

    _____

    b. Corrected statement: _____

    _____

    _____

2. The patient fell and hit her right arm and her head as she was standing up from her sofa.

    a. Heading: _____

    _____

    b. Underline Corrected statement: _____

_____

_____

3. The patient's doctor told us that result of the x-ray examination of the right arm was negative.

    a. Heading: _____

_____

    b. Corrected statement: _____

_____

_____

4. The patient lives in an apartment in an assisted living complex and meals, laundry services, and housekeeping services are provided, and she can get help with bathing as needed.

    a. Heading: _____

_____

    b. Corrected statement: _____

_____

_____

5. The patient told us that health care is "unneeded and usually dangerous."

    a. Heading: _____

_____

    b. Corrected statement: _____

_____

_____

PART IV. The following are the notes to yourself that you jotted down while reading the medical record and talking with a patient. The information is from an initial examination. (While jotting down notes for yourself, you did not consult Nursing Home XYZ's approved abbreviations list.)

Information from Reading the Medical Record

98 years old
female
family concerned and visits patient frequently
stopped walking during the past 2 weeks
refuses to walk now for nursing staff
referred by nursing with approval of house doctor, Dr. Frien
Caucasian
the patient has high blood pressure that is controlled by medication
no other medications
family history of high blood pressure
the patient does not smoke or drink

until a month ago, the patient had been very active in recreational activities, including arts and crafts, bingo, and social activities, with the recreational therapist

routine urinalysis was normal 1 wk. ago

Information from Part of the Examination of the Patient

says she has had arthritis in her knees for more than 50 years

says the arthritis in not the cause of her refusing to walk

has to go to the bathroom frequently to urinate

has used a wheelchair during the past 10 days to get around the nursing home

says she gets herself into her wheelchair without help

says she quit walking because she couldn't get to the bathroom in time when she stood up

says she keeps a towel in her wheelchair at the nursing home just in case she cannot control her bladder

has had some bladder control problems for about 5 years but they have become more severe in past few weeks

says she could not tell the doctor about her urinary problem because women are not supposed to talk with men about "those things"

says she doesn't know if it is possible to walk any more because her bladder control problem is so bad

says she has not told the nurses about it because the head nurse is male and she has beliefs about men and women talking about problems with urine

says she has not had any kind of treatment for her problem yet

says she has not walked in 10 days

says she wants to have this problem improved so that she can walk to the far wing of the nursing home to the recreational activities

says cannot push the wheelchair far enough to get to the recreational activities

Write this information into the History section of a note.

_____

_____

_____

_____

_____

_____

_____

_____

_____

_____

_____

_____

_____

_____

_____

_____

_____

_____

_____

_____

_____

_____

_____

_____

_____

_____

_____

_____

_____

_____

_____

_____

_____

_____

_____

_____

_____

_____

_____

_____

_____

_____

_____

_____

_____

_____

_____

_____

_____

_____

_____

_____

_____

_____

_____

_____

_____

_____

_____

_____

Answers to "Writing History: Worksheet 1" are provided in Appendix A.

PART I. In the following you will find the familiar headings used for the *History* part of the note. Each is followed by five blanks (more than are needed for the exercise). Below these headings are statements to be included in the note. Write the number of each in the blank following its appropriate heading. The statements you list after each heading should be in the order in which they would logically appear in a note (for instance, 1-5-3 may make more sense than if you were to order them 3-1-5). You may wish to write the note out on a separate piece of paper to assist yourself with this task.

A. <u>Demographics:</u> ____, ____ , ____ , ____ , ____

B. <u>Current Condition(s)/Chief Complaint(s):</u> ____, ____ , ____ , ____ , ____

C. <u>Social Hx:</u> ____, ____ , ____ , ____ , ____

D. <u>Employment/Work:</u> ____, ____ , ____ , ____ , ____

E. <u>Living Environment:</u> ____, ____ , ____ , ____ , ____

F. <u>General Health Status:</u> ____, ____ , ____ , ____ , ____

G. <u>Social/Health Habits:</u> ____, ____ , ____ , ____ , ____

H. <u>Family Hx:</u> ____, ____ , ____ , ____ , ____

I. <u>Medical/Surgical Hx:</u> ____, ____ , ____ , ____ , ____

J. <u>Functional Status/Activity Level:</u> ____, ____ , ____ , ____ , ____

K. <u>Medications:</u> ____, ____ , ____ , ____ , ____

L. <u>Other Clinical Tests:</u> ____, ____ , ____ , ____ , ____

1. Medical dx is fx (L) hip.
2. Walked for fitness every day prior to fx.
3. No significant medical/surgical hx.
4. House has 2 steps to enter c̄ no hand railing.
5. Ambulance took Pt. home from the hospital because Pt. cannot navigate steps c̄ walker.
6. Pt. c/o pain (L) hip when standing NWB (L) LE c̄ walker.
7. Lives c̄ husband.
8. Pt's parents died of heart disease.
9. Currently daughter has hired a baby sitter until Pt. recovers fully.
10. Husband is 79 y.o.
11. Pt. is 75 y.o. Asian-American female.
12. X-rays 1 wk. ago revealed fx (L) femoral neck.
13. Pt. is taking pain medication.
14. Pt's brother died of cancer at age 43.
15. Husband is home all of the time & can assist Pt. c̄ transfers as needed.
16. States health is good.
17. Denies medication for anything other than pain.
18. Describes 15 ft. from Pt's bed to toilet.
19. Denies hx of smoking.
20. Pt. is retired but provides day care services for her daughter's children.
21. Husband's back hurts when he assists Pt. c̄ transfers.
22. Only prior adm. to hospital was at time of daughter's birth.

23. Lives in a house that is on 1 level c̄ carpeted floor surfaces throughout.
24. Pt. also volunteers at a literacy program on Sat. mornings.
25. Husband helps with light housework duties & cooking s̄ difficulty.
26. Hx of drinking ~1 glass of wine/wk.

PART II. Mark the statements that should be places in the *History* category by placing an *H* on the line before the statement.

1. _____ Will refer to OT to assist c̄ dressing.
2. _____ DTRs WNL throughout LEs except diminished Ⓡ KJ.
3. _____ Amb training, beginning standing B/S & progressing to walker.
4. _____ Pt. goal is to amb. indep. c̄ walker 140 ft. × 3 within 2 wks.
5. _____ Pt. c/o pain Ⓡ foot c̄ amb. PWB c̄ a walker.
6. _____ AROM Ⓛ knee 0–90º.
7. _____ C/o itching & pulling in scar Ⓛ wrist.
8. _____ Rolls supine→side-lying Ⓡ c̄ max assist. of 1.
9. _____ Pt. wants to go to daughter's house until he no longer needs the walker.
10. _____ Rx @ B/S OD:
11. _____ Medical Hx: TIA in 2001, ASHD, CHF
12. _____ Dependent in transfers supine↔sit, sit↔stand, bed↔B/S chair.
13. _____ Pt. lives alone in a 2-story house; 5 steps c̄ handrail to enter.
14. _____ Pt. will be given written & verbal instruction in a HEP prior to D/C.
15. _____ Recommend home health care PT p̄ D/C.
16. _____ Pt. speaks very little English; speaks Spanish fluently.
17. _____ Skin in area of scar Ⓛ wrist is very taught & adhered to scar tissue.
18. _____ PTA Pt. exercised regularly.
19. _____ Pt. is oriented × 3.
20. _____ Education needs: safety, exercise program, ADL, use of devices/equipment, nature of condition, & the recovery process.

PART III. In the following you will find information that belongs in the *History* part of the note. A blank line precedes each statement. Following these History statements are the headings used in the History section of the note. Write the letter of the appropriate heading in the blank preceding each statement.

1. _____ The patient attends ABC Middle School and is in seventh grade.

2. _____ The patient was playing volleyball and she jumped up in the air and landed on her right hip.

3. _____ The patient's mother has a history of breast cancer and a right mastectomy in 1997 with no evidence of recurrence of the cancer.

4. _____ The patient has never used any kind of walker or cane or other assistive device before.

5. _____ The patient is taking meperidine HCl (Demerol) for pain.

6. _____ The patient is on the volleyball team at school and practices volleyball daily with the team.

7. _____ The patient is 13 years old.

8. _____ The house the patient lives in has three steps to enter the house with a handrail on the right side going up.

9. _____ The patient is right-handed.

10. _____ The patient has not experienced any major life changes during the past year.

11. _____ The patient has had no previous injuries or hospitalizations.

12. _____ The patient has a medical diagnosis of subcapital fracture right hip.

13. _____ The patient lives in a house with carpeted floor surfaces except for the kitchen.

14. _____ The x-ray examination shows a subcapital fracture in the right hip with a pin in place.

15. _____ The patient complains of "excruciating pain" in her right hip when she moves her right lower extremity at all.

16. _____ The patient's father has a history of hypertension that is controlled by medication.

17. _____ The patient's mother can assist the patient when she returns home.

18. _____ The patient and her mother rate the patient's general health as excellent.

19. _____ The patient is female.

20. _____ The patient says she does not have a history of alcohol or tobacco use.

21. _____ The patient's developmental history is within normal limits.

22. _____ The patient is Caucasian.

23. _____ The patient lives with her parents and an 11-year-old brother.

24. _____ There is a history of heart disease in the patient's maternal and paternal grandfathers.

25. _____ The patient was referred to physical therapy by Dr. Frume.

26. _____ The patient's mother does not work outside of the home.

27. _____ The patient's school has no steps.

28. _____ The laboratory test shows that the patient's hemoglobin value is 10.

29. _____ The patient has not been out of bed yet.

A. Demographics

B. Current Condition(s)/Chief Complaint(s)

C. Social Hx

D. School (substituting for Employment/Work)

E. Living Environment

F. General Health Status

G. Social/Health Habits

H. Family Hx

I. Development

J. <u>Medical/Surgical Hx</u>

K. <u>Functional Status/Activity Level</u>

L. <u>Medications</u>

M. <u>Other Clinical Tests</u>

PART IV. Write the preceding information into the History section of a note. Remember to use abbreviations and brevity in writing the note.

_____

_____

_____

_____

_____

_____

_____

_____

_____

_____

_____

_____

_____

_____

_____

_____

_____

_____

_____

_____

_____

_____

_____

_____

_____

_____

_____

_____

_____

_____

_____
_____
_____
_____
_____
_____
_____
_____
_____
_____
_____
_____
_____
_____
_____
_____
_____
_____
_____
_____
_____
_____
_____
_____
_____
_____
_____
_____
_____
_____
_____
_____
_____
_____
_____
_____
_____
_____
_____
_____

Answers to "Writing History: Worksheet 2" are provided in Appendix A.

The Patient/Client Management Format: Writing Systems Review

The *Systems Review* is the part of the Patient/ Client Management note that reports the results of a brief examination or screening of the cardiovascular/pulmonary, integumentary, musculoskeletal, and neuromuscular systems, and the patient's communication, affect, cognition, and learning style. This part of the note represents the first hands-on part of the examination. Except for the cardiovascular/pulmonary information, the information gathered in the Systems Review is reported as either *not impaired* or *impaired*. More specific descriptions and measurements are written in the Tests and Measures subsection of the Examination report.

After the Systems Review is completed, the therapist determines whether physical therapy is appropriate for the patient or whether the patient should be referred to another health practitioner, such as the patient's physician, or both. At times the Systems Review may not be completed because the therapist notes something from the patient's History and part of the Systems Review that indicates the patient needs to see another health care professional for care.

Categorizing Information in the Systems Review

An item belongs under Systems Review if any of the following apply:

- It involves basic Cardiovascular/Pulmonary information such as heart rate, respiratory rate, blood pressure, or edema. The Cardiovascular/ Pulmonary system is rated as *impaired or not impaired* as a whole system. Individual measurements of heart rate, blood pressure, respiratory rate, and a general description of edema are listed separately under this category.
Example: <u>Cardiovascular/Pulmonary System:</u> impaired. BP: 140/85. HR: 90 bpm. RR: 20. Edema: pitting edema noted bilat. ankles.

> ### E X A M P L E
>
> **Excerpts from the HISTORY section of the Examination and the SYSTEMS REVIEW:**
>
> **History:** <u>Current Condition:</u> Pt. c/o severe pain Ⓡ ankle and numbness & tingling in toes. Pt. states was injured at a softball game the night before & was sent home c̄ ankle wrapped in elastic wrap. States twisted ankle laterally and heard a "pop" at time of injury. Has iced and elevated ankle since injury. Called physician and was told to see physical therapist. <u>Other tests:</u> Pt. has not had an x-ray of Ⓡ ankle.
> **Systems Review:** <u>Cardiovascular/Pulmonary:</u> Severe edema noted Ⓡ ankle. <u>Integumentary:</u> Skin is stretched tight & is shiny in area of edema Ⓡ ankle. Toes are cold & blue.
> Pt.'s physician contacted & Pt. referred to ED for further care.

- It involves basic information on the Integumentary System such as integumentary disruption, continuity of skin color, skin pliability, or texture. The Integumentary System as a whole is listed as *impaired* or *not impaired*. Specific measurements are not reported in this section of the note, although basic information is listed.
Example: <u>Integumentary System:</u> impaired. Wound noted Ⓡ ant. leg. Skin discolored around area of wound. Skin thin & fragile bilat. LEs.

- It involves the basic information about the Musculoskeletal System such as gross symmetry during standing, sitting, and activities, gross range of motion, and gross muscle strength. The patient's height and weight are also recorded with musculoskeletal information. Specific range-of-motion and muscle testing is not reported in this section of the note. Each subcategory of

this section (gross symmetry, gross range of motion, gross muscle strength) is listed as *impaired* or *unimpaired*.
Example: <u>Musculoskeletal System:</u> gross symmetry: impaired in LEs in standing. Gross ROM: unimpaired bilat. LEs. Gross Strength: impaired bilat. LEs, Ⓡ > Ⓛ . Height: 5 ft. 6 in. Weight: 140 lbs.

● It involves the Neuromuscular System such as gait, locomotion (transfers, bed mobility), balance, and motor function (motor control, motor learning). Specific descriptions of these are not reported in this section of the note. Each individual subcategory (gait, locomotion, balance, motor function) under the Neuromuscular System is reported as *impaired* or *unimpaired*.
Example: <u>Neuromuscular System:</u> Gait unimpaired. Locomotion: transfers impaired. Balance: unimpaired. Motor function: unimpaired.

● It involves the patient's Communication Style or Abilities, including whether the patient's communication is age-appropriate. Specific communication abilities are reported as *impaired* or *unimpaired*.
Example: <u>Communication:</u> age appropriate & unimpaired.

● It involves the patient's Affect, such as the patient's emotional and behavioral responses. Specific affective abilities are reported as *impaired* or *unimpaired*.
Example: <u>Affect:</u> emotional/behavioral responses unimpaired.

● It involves the patient's Cognition, such as whether the patient is oriented to person, place, and time (oriented × 3) or the patient's level of consciousness. Cognitive abilities are reported as *impaired* or *unimpaired,* with specifics mentioned as necessary.
Example: <u>Cognition:</u> level of consciousness unimpaired. Orientation to person unimpaired; orientation to place & time impaired.

● It involves any Learning Barriers that the patient may have, such as vision, hearing, inability to read, inability to understand what is read, language barriers (needs for an interpreter), and any other learning barrier noted by the therapist. It should be noted that the use of glasses and hearing aids is listed in the *History* part of the note under Living Environment: Devices and Equipment. If the patient uses assistive devices that compensate for visual or hearing barriers, these barriers should only be noted if the assistive devices are not available, are not sufficient to compensate for the patient's learning barrier, or if

the patient requires additional assistance of some kind.
Example: <u>Learning Barriers:</u> hearing; Pt. understands best when able to see therapist's lips along with use of hearing aid.

● It involves the patient's Learning Style. This includes reporting how the patient or client best learns (pictures, reading, listening, demonstration, other).
Example: <u>Learning Style:</u> Pt. learns best when rationale for exercises is given before demonstration.

● It involves the patient's Education Needs. This includes reporting areas in which the patient needs more education or information, such as disease process, safety, use of devices or equipment, activities of daily living, exercise program, recovery and healing process and other education needs noted by the therapist. These are reported as a listing of all of the areas in which the patient needs education.
Example: <u>Education Needs:</u> disease process, home exercise program, use of the back in ADLs

Abbreviations and Medical Terminology

Appropriate use of abbreviations and medical terminology is expected, as well as correct spelling. Clarity and conciseness are important.

Categories Used to Report the Systems Review

The categories used in the *Systems Review* part of the note are very consistent. They are the following:

● Cardiovascular/Pulmonary

● Integumentary

● Musculoskeletal

● Neuromuscular

● Communication, Affect, Cognition, and Learning Style.

Information that is outside of the usual information in each of these categories can be written if it is outstanding and makes a difference in the therapist's decision to continue to examine a patient or to refer the patient elsewhere. In the example given previously, the therapist noted that the patient's toes were cold, although this was not a specific examination technique listed under the Integumentary System for Systems Review.

Writing Progress or Discharge Notes

Because the Systems Review is used for screening a patient for the appropriateness of therapy and the need to refer to other practitioners, this subsection of the note is generally not included in Progress or Discharge Notes.

Summary

The Systems Review Section of the Patient/Client Management note is the section in which the thera-pist performs some very basic general examination/screening techniques. This information helps the therapist to plan the rest of the examination and to decide whether the patient has a problem that physical therapy can treat. The categories or headings used in the Systems Review subsection of the note are consistent. The information recorded under these categories or headings should be written in a clear and concise manner and should use appropriate medical terminology and abbreviations.

The following worksheets give practice at the skills needed to write the Systems Review section of the note. After reviewing this chapter, working with the worksheets, and using the answer sheets to correct the worksheets, you will be able to write the Systems Review section of the note.

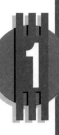

PART I. Mark the statements that should be placed under the Systems Review section of the note by placing an *SR* on the line before the statement. Also mark the History items with an *Hx*.

1. _____ Heart rate is 82 bpm.

2. _____ Gait is impaired.

3. _____ Pt. lives c̄ her mother & her son & his wife.

4. _____ Pt. has dx of Type I diabetes for 30 yrs.

5. _____ Oriented × 3.

6. _____ Pt. to be seen 2×/wk. in OP clinic.

7. _____ Gross AROM & PROM Ⓡ hip is impaired.

8. _____ Locomotion (transfers, bed mobility) is impaired.

9. _____ Pt. has htn controlled by medication.

10. _____ Pt. best learns through demonstration, practice c̄ cues, & then referral to pictures as memory cues.

11. _____ Medical dx is s/p AK amputation Ⓡ LE.

12. _____ Son's wife is able to drive Pt. to PT.

13. _____ Pliability of skin around scar is impaired.

14. _____ Pt. will amb. indep. c̄ prosthetic Ⓡ LE s assist. device p̄ 2 mo. of PT.

15. _____ No integumentary disruption noted; Ⓡ LE is healed.

16. _____ Communication is age-appropriate.

17. _____ Rx this date: teach Pt. home exercise program of stretching & strengthening to bilat. LEs & UEs.

18. _____ Pt. describes overall health as good.

19. _____ Education needs include use of prosthetic Ⓡ LE & assist. devices, safety, rehab. process, exercise program, ADLs.

20. _____ Balance standing: impaired.

PART II. Match each Systems Review statement with the appropriate heading. More than one statement may exist for each heading.

A. Cardiovascular/Pulmonary System
B. Integumentary System
C. Musculoskeletal System
D. Neuromuscular System
E. Communication, Affect, Cognition and Learning Style

1. _____ The patient requires a hearing aid to learn and communicate.

2. _____ The patient's height is 6 feet and 2 inches.

3. _____ The patient's gross muscle strength is impaired in the right upper extremity and is otherwise within normal limits.

4. _____ The patient's skin texture is thin and fragile.

5. _____ The patient's emotional and behavioral responses are impaired when the patient's breathing is more difficult.

6. _____ The patient's locomotion is impaired.

7. _____ The patient has multiple small tears in skin in the bilateral upper extremities.

8. _____ The patient's blood pressure is 130/83.

9. _____ The patient's heart rate is 92 beats per minute.

10. _____ The patient's balance is impaired.

11. _____ The patient's posture is impaired.

12. _____ The patient's gross active range of motion is impaired in the right upper extremity and otherwise is within normal limits.

13. _____ The patient weighs 180 pounds.

14. _____ The patient needs to learn about the disease process, the value of exercise, safety, and the use of adaptive equipment and assistive devices.

15. _____ The patient best learns from demonstration followed by reminders in the form of pictures.

16. _____ Inspection of the patient's skin color reveals multiple small hematomas noted below the skin.

17. _____ The patient's respiratory rate is 30.

18. _____ The patient's communication is age-appropriate.

19. _____ The patient's gait is impaired.

20. _____ The patient is oriented to person and place but is confused as to the date.

PART III. Using the categories and statements in Part II and using appropriate abbreviations and brevity, write the information into the Systems Review section of a note.

_____

_____

_____

_____

_____

_____

_____

_____

_____

_____

_____

Answers to "Writing Systems Review: Worksheet 1" are provided in Appendix A.

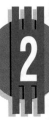

PART I. Mark each heading that belongs under the Systems Review section of the note by placing an *SR* on the line before the headings. Also mark the History headings with an *Hx.*

1. _____ Functional Status/Activity Level

2. _____ Neuromuscular System

3. _____ Demographic Information

4. _____ General Health Status

5. _____ Cardiovascular/Pulmonary System

6. _____ Medical/Surgical History

7. _____ Integumentary System

8. _____ Medications

9. _____ Social/Health Habits

10. _____ Communication, Affect, Cognition, Learning Style

12. _____ Social History

13. _____ Family History

14. _____ Other Clinical Tests

15. _____ Musculoskeletal System

16. _____ Current Conditions/Chief Complaint(s)

17. _____ Living Environment

PART II. Write the appropriate Systems Review Heading on the line before each statement below. As a reminder, Systems Review Standard Headings include Cardiovascular/Pulmonary System, Integumentary System, Musculoskeletal System, Neuromuscular System, Communication, Cognition, Affect, Language, Learning Style, and Education Needs.

1. _____ Blood pressure is 125/85.

2. _____ Heart rate is 80 beats per minute.

3. _____ Gross strength is impaired in both lower extremities.

4. _____ Height is 6 feet, 2 inches.

5. _____ Weight is 190 pounds.

6. _____ No scar tissue noted on either foot.

7. _____ Skin integrity is impaired. Open area noted on plantar surface of right foot.

8. _____ Gait is impaired.

9. _____ Respiratory rate is 13 breaths per minute.

10. _____ Communication is unimpaired.

11. _____ Skin color is impaired. It is red in the area surrounding the wound.

12. _____ Gross symmetry is impaired in lower extremities.

13. _____ Skin texture is impaired in both feet. It is thin and fragile.

14. _____ Gross range of motion is impaired in both feet and ankles.

15. _____ Oriented to person, place, time is unimpaired.

16. _____ Needs education in the disease process, safety, wound care, exercise program, activities of daily living, use of assistive devices, general foot care.

17. _____ Balance is impaired.

18. _____ Learns best by demonstration by therapist accompanied by home exercise program that includes illustrations.

19. _____ Does not wear glasses and sight is impaired as a result of cataracts.

20. _____ Locomotion is unimpaired.

21. _____ Emotional and behavioral responses are unimpaired.

22. _____ Edema noted in right foot surrounding the wound on the plantar surface.

PART III. Using the categories and statements in Part II, and using appropriate abbreviations and brevity, write the information into the Systems Review section of a note.

_____

_____

_____

_____

_____

_____

_____

_____

_____

_____

_____

_____

_____

_____

_____

_____

_____

_____

_____

_____

Answers to "Writing Systems Review: Worksheet 2" are provided in Appendix A.

The Patient/Client Management Format: Documenting Tests and Measures

The *Tests and Measures* is the section in which the results of tests and measures performed and the therapist's observations of the patient are recorded. It is located in the Examination section. Tests and measures are measurable or observable and contribute to the formation of the plan of care. Good tests and measures are repeatable, valid, and reliable. When tests and measures are recorded, the therapist can compare them with tests and measures recorded in the past. Tests and measures will serve as comparative data in the future, as the patient's progress is monitored and reevaluated. The effectiveness of therapeutic interventions can be evaluated using comparisons of tests and measures prior to and after the interventions are performed.

Categorizing Items into Tests and Measures

An item belongs in the Tests and Measures part of the Patient/Client Management note only if it is the result of a test performed by the therapist or an observation made by the therapist. Each profession has common tests and measures used by the profession for certain diagnoses.

EXAMPLE

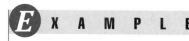

AROM: WNL throughout UEs & LEs except 120° ⓡ shoulder flexion noted.

Abbreviations and Medical Terminology

Appropriate use of abbreviations and medical terminology is expected, as is correct spelling.

The following pages discuss some methods of recording tests and measures. Use them as a reference. Clarity and conciseness are important.

Organization

Information should be organized, easy to read, and easy to find.

Categories

To organize the data from tests and measures better and make it easier to read, the data is divided into categories or headings. The headings or categories used depend on the patient's deficits and diagnosis.

Headings or categories can be based on the types of tests and measurements performed. This type of organization is helpful when the patient has deficits in several parts of the body or some type of generalized problem. Examples of categories include the following:

- Ambulation
- Transfers
- Balance
- Range of motion (ROM)
- Strength
- Sensation

Headings or categories can also be based on areas of the body and functional skills. Use of this type of organization is found when many of the patient's deficits are located in one or two parts of the body. Examples of categories include the following:

- Ambulation
- Activities of daily living (ADLs)
- Independent activities of daily living (IADLs)
- Upper extremities (UEs)
- Lower extremities (LEs)
- Trunk

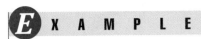

Poorly Written

TESTS AND MEASURES: UE Strength 5/5 except triceps. Amb c̄ standard walker NWB (R) LE ≈ 2 ft. × 1 c̄ mod. assist of 1. (L) LE: Strength 5/5 except for gluteal musculature. Vital signs 3 min. p̄ amb.: BP: 125/80, HR: 85, RR: 14. 4/5 triceps strength noted bilat. Able to manage NWB status (R) LE indep. 3+/5 (L) gluteus maximus & gluteus medius noted. (R) musculature controlling knee & ankle not tested this date 2° long leg cast. Transfers sit ↔ stand c̄ min. assist. of 1. (R) LE strength at hip 5/5 except gluteal musculature. Vitals @ rest: BP 125/82, HR: 80, RR: 13. Transfers w/c ↔ bed c̄ mod. assist of 1. Able to wiggle toes (R) LE; further testing deferred 2° recent trimalleolar fx. Transfers supine ↔ sit c̄ min. assist. of 1. 3+/5 (R) gluteus maximus & gluteus medius noted. Vital signs immed. p̄ amb.: BP 140/85, HR: 120, RR: 20. Transfers on/off toilet c̄ mod. assist of 1.

Properly Written

TESTS AND MEASURES: Amb: c̄ standard walker NWB (R) LE ≈2 ft. × 1 c̄ mod. assist of 1. ADLs: transfers sit ↔ stand & supine ↔ sit c̄ min. assist. of 1. Transfers w/c ↔ bed & on/off toilet c̄ mod. assist. of 1. UEs: Strength 5/5 except 4/5 triceps noted. (L) LE: Strength: 5/5 except 3+/5 gluteus maximus & gluteus medius. (R) LE: Strength at hip 5/5 except 3+/5 gluteus maximus & gluteus medius. Musculature controlling knee & ankle not tested this date 2° long leg cast. Able to wiggle toes; further testing deferred 2° recent trimalleolar fx. Able to manage NWB status indep. Aerobic capacity & endurance: Vitals @ rest: BP 125/82, HR: 80, RR: 13; vital signs immed. p̄ amb.: BP 140/85, HR: 120, RR: 20; vital signs 3 min. p̄ amb.: BP: 125/80, HR: 85, RR: 14.

The following are also examples of categories:

- Ambulation
- ADLs
- IADLs
- (R) Extremities
- (L) Extremities
- Trunk

Use of categories varies from one clinical facility to another. Certain facilities require therapists to categorize information on all patients in the same manner despite differences between patients in diagnoses and deficits. (For example, all notes in one facility might have the categories *gait, ADL, IADL, strength, ROM,* and *sensation.*) This may be done to compare data across similar cases. Other facilities give the therapists more freedom to categorize information in the manner they deem most efficient and organized. For the purposes of this workbook, you are expected to choose the most appropriate categories for each patient's specific diagnosis and deficits.

Within the *Tests and Measures* portion of a note, the categories can be arranged using a number of different methods. Some clinicians list the functional activities (gait, transfers, ADL) first because they believe that functional activities are the most important. Others believe that the impairments should be listed first because specific information on impairments is needed to understand the reasons for functional deficits. Most of the audiences for patient care notes (physicians, insurance reviewers, lawyers, utilization reviewers, and social workers) prefer listing the functional activities first, with the impairments listed after the functional deficits. For the purposes of this workbook, you are expected to address functional activities and deficits before listing impairments.

Within any individual category in the *Tests and Measures* subsection of a note, the information is organized in the most logical order possible. Usually one joint at a time is described, and joints are addressed from proximal to distal. Information is otherwise grouped as efficiently as possible within this framework.

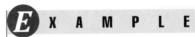

TESTS & MEASURES: UEs: AROM: WNL except for 80° (R) shoulder flexion & 90° (R) elbow flexion. STRENGTH: 4–/5 throughout (R) shoulder musculature, 4+/5 biceps, 4/5 triceps, 3/5 musculature controlling the wrist & fingers. SENSATION: Intact throughout.

Methods of Recording Data from Tests and Measures

In many facilities, complete sentences are not necessary, but information should be clear enough to get the idea across.

E X A M P L E

Unclear

AROM: ankle in cast.

Clear

AROM: Ⓛ ankle not tested 2° short leg cast Ⓛ LE.

At times, using a table format gets the information across in the most complete manner.

E X A M P L E

Strength: Comparison of strength of LEs is as follows:

Musculature	Ⓛ LE	Ⓡ LE
Hip	5/5 all musculature	5/5 all musculature
Quadriceps	3/5	5/5
Hamstrings	2/5	5/5
Ankle and foot	0/5 all musculature except 1/5 anterior tibialis	5/5 all musculature

Sometimes a standard ROM or muscle testing chart, flow sheet, or some other standardized table can be used (many therapy departments have these available for use). Instead of giving detailed information within the note, the therapist can refer to the flow sheet or table and attach a copy to the note.

E X A M P L E

Strength: LEs: See attached table; limited Ⓛ LE.

A table or flow sheet should always be dated and signed and include the patient's name and medical record number.

Common Mistakes in Recording Data from Tests and Measures

Some of the most common mistakes in recording data from tests and measures are the following:

- Failure to state the affected body part
- Failure to state measurable information
- Failure to state the type of whatever it is that is being measured or observed

E X A M P L E

Correct
- *AROM*, the type of ROM measured
- Shoulder *flexion*, the type of movement measured
- *Gait* deviations, the type of deviations observed
- *Sliding board w/c → mat* transfers, the type of transfers observed

Writing Progress Notes

In a progress note, not every category addressed in an initial note is included. Use only the information obtained while re-examining the patient during treatment sessions. However, keep in mind that any test and measure describing a functional deficit or impairment in the initial note should be re-examined and addressed in an interim note in the future.

If a patient's status is unchanged and the area addressed is extremely important, it is acceptable to address the area and state that it is unchanged. However, for the sake of the reader, the unchanged status should be briefly described.

E X A M P L E

Correct

Transfers: Supine → sit unchanged; still requires mod assist of 1.

When stating that the patient's status is unchanged, it is important to make sure that all of the tests and measures available have been used. In the previous example, perhaps the amount of assistance needed by the patient is unchanged, but the patient is performing the transfer more quickly (2 minutes to perform the transfer versus 5 minutes).

E X A M P L E

Better

Transfers: Supine → sit unchanged; still requires mod assist. of 1 but performance of transfer requires 2 min. on this date (vs. 5 min. initially required). Transfer is becoming more functional.

Data used for comparison purposes can also be included. In the previous example, without the comparative data, the fact that the performance of the transfer required 2 minutes would seem insignificant to the reader. The reader may not take the time to look at a previously written note to obtain the patient's former status, or the reader may not have the previous note available.

Information addressed in progress notes should include areas addressed in the last set of anticipated goals written. For example, if a goal is set for the patient to be able to roll supine → sidelying independently within 1 week, the patient's rolling status should be addressed in the Tests and Measures subsection in the next progress note.

▌Writing Discharge Notes

The completeness of the Tests and Measures subsection of a discharge note varies greatly among practice settings. In some facilities, the discharge note is similar to an interim note and is an update of the patient's status since the last interim note was written. In other facilities, the discharge note is a more complete summary of the patient's condition upon discharge from the facility. In these facilities, the Tests and Measures subsection of the note may list all of the functional deficits noted in the initial note with the progress from the initial note to discharge listed. The same may be true for impairments listed in the initial note, depending on the progress made.

Types of notes can also vary depending on who will be reading the note. For example, a note that is forwarded to a nursing home or home health agency might be a complete summary of the patient's condition, whereas a note that will go the medical records storage when the patient is discontinued may simply update the patient's status since the last interim note was written. The home health therapist or nursing home therapist may receive only the discharge summary from an acute or rehabilitation facility, so a more complete note is needed. For the purposes of this workbook, the discharge note is considered a complete summary of the patient's status on discharge and course of therapy, and you are to address all tests and measures used during the course of the patient's care.

▌Summary

The Tests and Measures subsection of the note is a very important section. It should be included in every note, whether it is an initial, progress, or discharge note. The information should be organized under headings, should be written in a clear and concise manner, and should list the results of tests and measures performed by the therapist.

The following worksheets give practice at the skills needed to write the Tests and Measures subsection of a note. After reviewing this chapter, working through the following worksheets, and using the answer sheets to correct the worksheets, you should be able to write accurately the Tests and Measures subsection of a note.

Documenting Tests and Measures:

Worksheet 1

PART I. On the blank line to the left of each statement, mark the statements that should be placed in the Tests and Measures subsection by placing *TM* on the line before the statement. Also mark the History items with an *Hx* and the information that belongs in the Systems Review subsection of the note by writing *SR*.

1. _____ DTRs 2+ throughout LEs except 3+ ⓡ KJ.

2. _____ Pt. was in a car accident & Pt.'s car was hit broadside on the passenger side.

3. _____ Will refer Pt. to OT to assist c̄ dressing.

4. _____ <u>Expected Outcome</u>: Indep. walker amb 150 ft. × 2 FWB within 2 wks.

5. _____ Amb. training, beginning in // bars & progressing to a walker, emphasizing normal wt. distribution on LEs bilat.

6. _____ Strength testing inconsistent because Pt. does not follow commands to hold against resistance.

7. _____ <u>Learning Barriers</u>: none noted

8. _____ C/o inability to dress indep.

9. _____ <u>Transfers</u>: Supine ↔ sit c̄ min. assist of 1.

10. _____ <u>X-ray</u>: Osteoporosis throughout lumbar spine.

11. _____ ↑ PROM ⓛ knee to 0–90° within 2 wks.

12. _____ <u>Cognition:</u> Impaired; oriented to person only.

13. _____ <u>Proprioception:</u> ↓ throughout ⓡ UE.

14. _____ C/o pain throughout ⓛ UE c̄ passive movement of the wrist.

15. _____ AROM ⓡ shoulder flexion: ↑ to 0–90° p̄ Rx.

16. _____ Will be seen BID @ B/S:

17. _____ Pt. will be given written & verbal instructions in walking program & home exercise program for ⓡ UE strengthening.

18. _____ <u>Sensation:</u> Absent to light touch & pinprick through ⓛ L5 distribution.

19. _____ Pt. will demonstrate proper knowledge of back care & ADL p̄ discussion of ADLs & IADLs c̄ therapist & through 90% correct performance on an obstacle course for back ADLs & IADLs.

20. _____ C/o itching in scar ⓛ wrist ≈2×/hr.

PART II. Match each Tests and Measures statement with the appropriate heading. More than one statement may exist for each heading. Place the answer on the first blank line to the left of each statement.

A. Amb
B. ADL
C. UEs
D. LEs
E. Trunk

1. _____ LE AROM is WNL bilat except SLR bilat limited to 0–50° due to tight hamstrings.

_____

2. _____ Transfers supine ↔ sit indep but slow; requires 2 minutes to perform transfer.

_____

3. _____ Spasm noted Ⓛ lower lumbar paraspinal musculature.

_____

4. _____ LE strength is WNL bilat except 3/5 Ⓛ plantar flexors.

_____

5. _____ Tenderness to palpation in L4–5, L5–S1 area.

_____

6. _____ Pain in back increased to 8 & centralized to L4–5, L5–S1 area c̄ prone ext exercises; Ⓛ LE pain 0 (0–10 scale used).

_____

7. _____ UE AROMs & strengths WNL.

_____

8. _____ Trunk AROM is WNL; repeated flexion in standing & supine positions ↑ pain in low back & Ⓛ LE.

_____

9. _____ Posture: ↓ lumbar lordosis, head held in forward position, ↑ thoracic kyphosis.

_____

10. _____ Amb is indep s̄ device is slow c̄ little trunk rotation noted; amb. 30 ft. in 1 min.

_____

11. _____ Ankle jerk 1+ on Ⓛ, 2+ on Ⓡ.

_____

12. _____ SLR: + at 45° Ⓛ, − on Ⓡ.

_____

13. _____ Demonstrates improper lifting techniques when asked to lift a box & when asked to transfer Pts.

_____

14. _____ LE sensation to light touch & pinprick is diminished in Ⓡ L5 dermatome; otherwise WNL.

_____

15. _____ Repeated trunk extension in standing ↓ pain.

_____

PART III. On the second blank to the left of each of the previous statements, mark whether the Tests and Measures statement discusses function (write Func on the line) or a physical impairment (write Impair on the line).

PART IV. The following are the notes to yourself that you jotted down while performing the tests and measures part of your examination. (While taking notes for yourself, you did not consult Hospital XYZ's approved abbreviations list.)

1. sit ↔ stand minimal +1 assist
2. // bars—stood minimal +1 assist—1 min. twice then took 1 step c̄ minimal +1—FWB both LEs
3. LE strength at least 3/5 (group muscle test)—unable to further test due to mental status
4. UE strength at least 3/5 (group muscle test)—unable to test further due to mental status
5. all ROM WNL except approximately 90° shoulder abduction & approximately 110 degrees shoulder flexion bilaterally
6. fatigued after standing twice, all other examination deferred

Place an "X" before the headings you would use to write the Tests and Measures portion of this note.

_____ UEs

_____ LEs

_____ trunk

_____ transfers

_____ amb

_____ activity tolerance

_____ strength

_____ AROM

_____ Ⓡ extremities

_____ ADL

_____ Ⓛ extremities

PART V. Following, you will find headings for the Tests and Measures portion of the note. (These headings were chosen because they require the least repetition.) Each heading is followed by five blanks (more than are needed for the exercise). Using the notes you wrote previously, write the number of each after its appropriate heading. The information you list after each heading should be in the order in which information would logically appear in a note (for instance, 1-5-3 may make more sense than if you were to order them 3-1-5).

A. Amb: ____, ____ , ____ , ____ , ____

B. Transfers: ____, ____ , ____ , ____ , ____

C. Strength: ____, ____ , ____ , ____ , ____

D. AROM: ____, ____ , ____ , ____ , ____

E. Activity tolerance: ____, ____ , ____ , ____ , ____

PART VI. Using the categories listed in Part VI, write the information into the Tests and Measures portion of a note. Your partial note should be written to be an acceptable part of the patient's medical record at Hospital XYZ (using approved abbreviations).

TESTS & MEASURES: _____

_____

_____

_____

_____

_____

_____

_____

_____

_____

_____

_____

_____

_____

_____

_____

_____

_____

_____

_____

_____

_____

_____

Answers to "Tests and Measures: Worksheet 1" are provided in Appendix A.

Documenting Tests and Measures:
Worksheet 2

PART I. In the following you will find familiar headings discussed for the Tests and Measures portion of an interim note. Each heading is followed by five blanks (more than are needed for the exercise). Below these headings are seven statements to be included in the note. Write the number of each after its appropriate heading. The statements you list after each heading should be in the order in which they would logically appear in a note (for instance, 1-5-3 may make more sense than if you were to order them 3-1-5). You may wish to write the note out on a separate piece of paper to assist you with this task.

A. Gait: ____, ____ , ____ , ____ , ____

B. Transfers: ____, ____ , ____ , ____ , ____

C. Strength: ____, ____ , ____ , ____ , ____

1. Sit → stand $\bar{c}$ min +1 assist. & verbal cues for hand placement.
2. Stand → sit $\bar{c}$ mod +1 assist.; pt. does not reach for chair $\bar{a}$ attempting to sit.
3. Amb 100 ft × 3 $\bar{c}$ walker & min +1 assist.
4. Sit → supine $\bar{c}$ standby assist. of 1 & verbal cues.
5. Supine → sit $\bar{c}$ mod assist. of 1.
6. Bilat LE strength grossly 4–/5.
7. Has difficulty turning $\bar{c}$ walker.

PART II. The following is a note written by a student. Using the same information, rewrite this Tests and Measures portion of the note using different categories and more concise writing, if and when possible.

TESTS & MEASURES: <u>Appearance:</u> Incision Ⓡ anterior forearm covered $\bar{c}$ steri-strips. <u>AROM:</u> Ⓡ UE limited shoulder flexion to approx. 120°, abduction to approx. 70°, full elbow flexion, −42° elbow extension, full wrist flexion, wrist extension to neutral $\bar{c}$ full finger flexion. Ⓛ UE full AROM all movements. LEs full AROM all movements. <u>Strength</u> (gross break test used): Ⓡ UE shoulder flexion 3+, shoulder abduction 3+, elbow flexion & extension 4, wrist flexion/extension 4, finger flexion & extension 4. Ⓛ UE 5/5 all movements. Ⓛ LE 4 all movements. Ⓡ LE normal all movements. <u>Sensation:</u> To light touch & pinprick normal all 4 extremities. <u>Transfers:</u> W/c ↔ mat pivot transfer $\bar{c}$ minimal assist. of 1, sit ↔ supine indep. <u>Ambulation:</u> $\bar{c}$ walker $\bar{c}$ minimal assist for 50 ft. once wt. bearing as tolerated all extremities.

TESTS & MEASURES: _____

_____

_____

_____

_____

_____

_____

_____

Answers to "Writing Tests & Measures: Worksheet 2" are provided in Appendix A.

Review Worksheet:

Writing the History, Systems Review, and Tests and Measures

PART I. Indicate which of the following statements belong in the *History, Systems Review,* and Tests and Measures sections of the Patient/Client Management note. Mark them by placing an *Hx, SR* or *TM* on the blank line before the appropriate statement. (Some of the statements do not belong in the Examination part of the note.)

1. _____ Incision healing well, length 3 in. location immediately prox. to Ⓛ thumb-nail.

2. _____ ↑AROM Ⓡ shoulder to WNL within 4 wks. c̄ 3×/wk. Rx.

3. _____ Will instruct Pt. in a home exercise program to improve posture & alignment (attached).

4. _____ Pt's wife states he amb indep s̄ assist. device PTA.

5. _____ DTRs: 2+ throughout.

6. _____ Medical dx: low back pain.

7. _____ Past experience of PT for low back pain s̄ relief of pain.

8. _____ C/o Ⓡ LE pain in posterolateral aspects of Ⓡ thigh down to the knee; pain intensity: 8 (0 = no pain, 10 = worst possible pain).

9. _____ Will attempt to perform manual muscle test on another date when Pt. is more rested.

10. _____ X-ray: arthritic spurs L3–5 Ⓡ.

11. _____ HR: 75 ā exercise, 95 immediately p̄ exercise, & 75 bpm 3 min. p̄ exercise.

12. _____ Amb s̄ assist. device indep & s̄ deviations

13. _____ Describes onset of pain immed. p̄ lifting a 50 lb. bag of dog food on 01/01/20XX.

14. _____ BID: hot pack to low back for 20 min.

15. _____ Pt's rehab. potential is guarded.

PART II. Rewrite the following History, Systems Review, and Tests and Measures statements in a more clear, concise, and professional manner. Also, list the subsection of the notes (History, Systems Review, or Tests and Measures) and the heading under which the statement should be placed.

1. The patient complains of the left lateral knee pain that comes and goes.

   a. <u>Part of the note:</u> _____

   b. <u>Heading:</u> _____

   c. <u>Corrected statement:</u> _____

2. The patient doesn't have as much sensation in the left L5 dermatome.

    a. <u>Part of the note:</u> _____

    b. <u>Heading:</u> _____

    c. <u>Corrected statement:</u> _____

3. The patient states a doctor "looked in [his] right knee with a scope" on 02/02/2003.

    a. <u>Part of the note:</u> _____

    b. <u>Heading:</u> _____

    c. <u>Corrected statement:</u> _____

4. The patient says he had "surgery where they opened up my skull" in February 2003.

    a. <u>Part of the note:</u> _____

    b. <u>Heading:</u> _____

    c. <u>Corrected statement:</u> _____

5. Right leg passive range of motion is within normal limits throughout.

    a. <u>Part of the note:</u> _____

    b. <u>Heading:</u> _____

    c. <u>Corrected statement:</u> _____

PART III. Here are the notes to yourself that you jotted down while reading the chart and examining your patient. (While taking notes for yourself, you did not consult Hospital XYZ's approved abbreviations, list.)

From the Chart

Diagnosis is fractured right femoral neck on 01/12/2003. A right hip prosthesis was inserted on 01/13/2003. Patient is 65 years old. The patient is male. Physician is Dr. Sosome. Hgb was 11 this morning. You are seeing the patient on 01/15/2003. You tried to see the patient on 01/14/2003 but patient was dizzy lying in bed and Hgb was 7. Patient received blood transfusion on 01/14/2003.

From the Patient

Pain Ⓡ hip while standing 8/10, while lying (before ambulation) 4/10
No PT or OT before—no walker or cane before this admission—no tub chair or portable commode currently available at home—no other assistive devices used for dressing, bathing, ambulating
Fell at home and hit Ⓡ hip on side of bathtub
Lives alone—senior apartment building—elevator—curbs only
Apartment bathroom has a bathtub with a shower and shower curtain
Retired this year—was a teacher—still volunteers at elementary school 3 days per week, reading with small children
For recreation, patient watches her grandchildren and plays cards with friends. Watches toddler-aged grandchildren once per week and plays cards with friends 2 nights per week.
Would like to return to her apartment after discharge
(For PTs:) Would like to eventually ambulate independently s̄ device once again

(For OTs:) Would like to able to manage grooming and dressing by herself; would "settle" for
    Meals on Wheels
Walks approximately 2 miles 3 times per week
Does not drink alcohol and does not smoke

Systems Review

Blood pressure was 140/80
Initially pulse rate was 80
Respiratory rate was 12
Neuromuscular system: gait impaired, locomotion impaired, balance impaired in standing
    and during ambulation, motor function unimpaired
Integumentary system: impaired at surgery site; otherwise WNL
Musculoskeletal system: gross strength impaired on the right as is the range of motion
Communication is unimpaired
Affect: the patient's emotional/behavioral responses are unimpaired
Cognition: oriented to person, place and time, unimpaired
Learning barriers: patient wears glasses and cannot read without them—therefore, will need
    them for the home exercise program
Learning style—likes to be shown by the therapist and then tries to imitate therapist's
    actions—visual learner
Education needs—needs to learn how to use a walker on level surfaces and on curbs, needs to
    learn transfers, needs to learn to check for proper healing of wound, needs a home exer-
    cise program

PT Examination Performed

UEs—ROMs WNL except –5 degrees of right elbow extension
UEs—strength 4+/5 throughout (group muscle test)
ROMs in left leg WNL
Right LE—ROMs limited secondary to post-op restrictions to 90° hip flexion, full active hip
    abduction, 0° hip medial and lateral rotation, 0° adduction
Left LE—strength 4+/5 throughout (group muscle tests)
Right LE—strength at least 3/5 throughout—not further examined due to recent surgery
Transfers   w/c to and from bed c̄ moderate of 1 person
               Sit to and from stand with minimal of 1 person
               Supine to and from sit with moderate of 1 person
Ambulated—parallel bars minimal of 1 approximately 20 feet once 50% PWB right LE—felt
    dizzy and nauseated—no further examination or interventions performed this date—
    nurses notified
BP: 145/90 immediately after ambulation, 135/80 3 min. after ambulation
Pulse 105 immediately after ambulation, 82 3 min. after ambulation
Breathing rate: 18 immediately after ambulation; 12 3 minutes after ambulation

OT examination performed

UE strength 4+/5 throughout (group muscle test)
UE—AROM WNL except –5 degrees right elbow extension
Fine motor skills within normal limits
Transfers supine to and from sit with moderate assistance of 1
Transfers wheelchair to and from bed with moderate of 1
Patient initially seen bedside for assessment of grooming and dressing skills
Currently has IV infusing in left forearm
Patient able to bathe UE and trunk but needs minimal assistance of 1 for both LEs and
    needs setup for sponge bath

Able to groom his hair independently
Able to care for his teeth independently
Wears contact lenses; able to care for lenses by himself from a wheelchair
Dressing not assessed this date due to high pain level and low patient endurance

Write the preceding information into the History, Systems Review, and Tests and Measures portions of either a physical therapy note or an occupational therapy note. Your partial note should be written to be an acceptable part of the patient's medical record at Hospital XYZ.

_____
_____
_____
_____
_____
_____
_____
_____
_____
_____
_____
_____
_____
_____
_____
_____
_____
_____
_____
_____
_____
_____
_____
_____
_____

Answers to Review Worksheet: History, Systems Review and Tests and Measures can be found in Appendix A.

The SOAP Note:
Stating the Problem

The *Problem or Diagnosis* is the first section of the SOAP note. While learning how to write in the SOAP note format, you will notice you are using the same information that you used to write in the Patient/Client Management Note format but you are organizing according to the source of the information instead of the type of information.

In many facilities, the major problem or problems that have brought the patient to you for treatment are stated before actually beginning the SOAP note itself. This is usually stated as *Problem* or *Dx*. The Problem part of the note can be stated as the patient's chief complaint, the diagnosis, or a loss of function. It may be medical, psychological, or functional.

In some facilities the pertinent history or medical information taken from the chart is included in the Problem area. In others it is the first information written in the Objective part of the note. For the purposes of this workbook, you are expected to state this information in the Problem area of the note, because it is not the result of tests you have conducted (your interview or measurements). Information such as the following is included:

- **Recent or past surgeries** affecting the present condition or treatment (e.g., hx of Ⓡ total knee replacement performed on [date]).

- **Past conditions/diseases** affecting the present condition or treatment (e.g., hx of CVA in 2001).

- **Present conditions/diseases** affecting the present condition or treatment (e.g., hypertension, CHF).

- **Medical test results** affecting the present condition or treatment (e.g., x-ray reveals fx Ⓛ tibial plateau).

Examples of the Problem part of the note are as follows:

1. <u>Dx</u>:Ⓛhemiplegia resulting from craniotomy for removal of tumor on 09-12-20XX. Hx of htn. Referring physician: Dr. Alexad.
2. 58-yr.-old ♂ c̄ ⓁBK amputation on 02-17-2003 2° PVD. Hx of diabetes. Referring physician: Dr. Ollandern.

There are no worksheets on writing the problem. As you practice writing notes on the worksheets that follow, you are expected to state the problem (if it is given to you) before you write the rest of the note. You will get much practice at stating the problem in completing this workbook.

The SOAP Note: Writing Subjective (S)

The *Subjective* part of the note is the section in which the therapist is able to state the information received from the patient that is relevant to the patient's present condition. Subjective information is necessary to plan the objective assessment of the patient and to justify or explain certain goals that are set with the patient. For example, third-party payers, utilization review auditors, and quality assurance auditors may question testing a patient's ability to go up and down a flight of 16 steps or teaching a patient to go up and down those steps (and why it is taking the patient longer than other patients his age to become independent) unless the Subjective part of the note includes documentation that the patient has 16 steps to enter his home.

Categorizing Items as Subjective

An item belongs in the Subjective category if any of the following apply:

- *The patient* (or significant other) tells the therapist or assistant about the patient's **current conditions/chief complaints.** This includes the onset date of the problem, any incident that caused or contributed to the onset of the problem, prior history of similar problems, how the patient is caring for the problem, what makes the problem better and worse, and any other health care provider the patient is seeing for the problem.

- *The patient* (or significant other) tells the therapist or assistant about the activities that the patient can no longer perform as a result of the patient's current condition. This includes information on everything from bed mobility, transfers, gait, self-care, home management, to community and work activities that apply to the patient's current situation or condition. This is often referred to as **functional status/activity level** of the patient.

- *The patient* (or significant other) tells the therapist or assistant about his or her cultural and religious beliefs that might affect care, the person(s) with whom the patient lived prior to admission and will live with at discharge, available social and physical supports the patient has now and will have at discharge, and the availability of a caregiver. This is referred to as **social history.**

- *The patient* (or significant other) tells the therapist or assistant whether he or she works full time or part time, inside or outside of the home, is retired or is a student. This is referred to as **employment status.**

- *The patient* (or significant other) tells the therapist or assistant the devices and equipment the patient uses; the type of residence in which the patient lives; information about the living environment such as stairs or ramps available; and past use of community services, including day services and programs, home health services, homemaking services, hospice, Meals on Wheels, mental health services, respiratory therapy, or rehabilitation therapy (physical therapy, occupational therapy, speech-language pathology). This is referred to as **living environment.**

- *The patient* (or significant other) tells the therapist or assistant about the patient's **general health status.** This includes a rating of the patient's health and whether the patient has experienced any major life changes during the past year.

- *The patient* (or significant other) tells the therapist or assistant about the patient's past and current **social/health habits,** such as alcohol and tobacco use and exercise habits.

- *The patient* (or significant other) tells the therapist or assistant about the patient's **family health history.** This is a general screening for a family history of heart disease, hypertension, stroke, diabetes, cancer, psychological conditions, arthritis, osteoporosis, and other conditions.

- *The patient* (or significant other) tells the therapist or assistant about the patient's **medical/surgical history.**

- *The patient* (or significant other) tells the therapist or gives the therapist a list of all of the **medications** the patient takes.

- *The patient* (or significant other) tells the therapist about the **growth and development** of the patient. This includes the developmental history of a patient and is most applicable to pediatric patients.

- *The patient* (or significant other) tells the therapist about **other clinical tests** applicable to the patient's current condition that the patient has experienced, such as laboratory tests or radiologic tests and the dates and findings of those tests.

- *The patient* reports a **response to treatment interventions** (e.g., a decrease in pain intensity).

- *The patient* tells the therapist the **patient's goals** for therapy.

- **Anything** *the patient* (or a designated significant other) tells the therapist or assistant that is relevant and significant to the patient's case or present condition.

The relevant history and other relevant information regarding the patient that is obtained from the chart may be stated under the Problem section (in some facilities, it is stated under the O, Objective, section). It does not belong under the Subjective section because it is not something that the patient (or significant other) tells the therapist directly.

Use of the Term *Patient*

Generally, the *S* section of the note should be as brief (yet complete) as possible. It is acceptable to use "Pt." the first time, but do not repeat it with every sentence. It is assumed, unless otherwise stated, that the information in this section came from the patient.

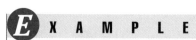 **X A M P L E**

Incorrect: Pt. c/o pain in Ⓡ low back area. Pt. states pain ↓'s c̄ rest. Pt. states is unable to work or perform most ADLs because pt. cannot sit >5 min. 2° pain.
This is a waste of time and space!

Correct: Pt. c/o pain in Ⓡ low back area. States pain ↓'s c̄ rest; is unable to work or perform most ADLs because cannot sit >5 min. 2° pain.

Abbreviations and Medical Terminology

Appropriate abbreviations and use of medical terminology are expected. Correct spelling is necessary for the therapist to be represented appropriately as a professional. The most concise (yet complete) wording should be used. Full sentences are not necessary if the idea is complete (this varies from facility to facility).

 X A M P L E

Wordy: The pt. states pain began ~3 wks. ago Wed.

More concise: Pt. states onset of pain on (date).

Organization

It is important for the sake of the other professionals reading the note to organize the note by topic. Often, subcategories, or headings, such as *current conditions/chief complaints, functional status/activity level, social history, employment status, living environment, general health status, social/health habits, family health history, medical/surgical history, medications, growth and development, other clinical tests, patient goals,* and *response to treatment interventions* are used. To which of the two examples in the following would you rather refer if you were looking for particular information?

 X A M P L E

1. Pt. c/o pain Ⓡ ankle when Ⓡ ankle is in a dependent position. Lives alone & must prepare all meals. Pt.'s goal is to play basketball again. Denies previous use of crutches. Denies any other pain or dizziness. Describes 3 steps s̄ a handrail at entrance to his home. States hx of a fall at home & feeling his Ⓡ ankle "pop." States played basketball 3×/wk. PTA.

2. Current condition: c/o pain Ⓡ ankle when Ⓡ ankle is in a dependent position. Denies any other pain or dizziness. States fell at home & felt his Ⓡ ankle "pop." Living environment: Describes 3 steps s̄ a handrail at entrance to his home. Denies use of crutches PTA. Social/health habits: States played basketball 3×/wk. PTA. Patient goals: Pt.'s goal is to play basketball again.

In the first example, getting a clear picture of the patient's status is difficult. The second example is much easier to read.

Almost every note should include information on the patient's *Current condition/chief complaint, functional status/activity level,* and *patient goals.* Initial notes should also include the other categories listed previously because that information is needed for clinical decision-making and discharge planning.

Do not include information or subcategories in the *S* section of the note just for the sake of inclusion. The purpose of information included in any part of the note is to address the patient's present condition and problems accurately and to assist in monitoring progress, revising the patient's program, and discontinuing therapy when necessary. Information that is not relevant to the patient's present condition, levels of functioning, or need for function at home should not be included. Irrelevant information wastes time, makes the note unnecessarily long, and may confuse all those who read the chart for purposes of case management, quality care assessment, discharge planning, utilization review, or reimbursement. For further information on reimbursement issues, see Appendix D.

▌ Verbs

S statements frequently contain a verb that indicates that the statement is subjective and not taken from the chart. Verbs frequently used are *states, describes, denies, indicates, c/o.*

▌ Quoting the Patient Verbatim

At times, quoting the patient verbatim is the most appropriate method of conveying subjective information. Some reasons for using direct quotes from the patient or a family member include the following:

- To illustrate **confusion** or **memory loss.** (Example: Pt. frequently states, "My mother will make everything all right. I want my mother." Pt. is 80 years old.) This can be used to illustrate why progress is slow or why therapy interventions may be inappropriate at this time.

- To illustrate **denial.** (Example: Pt.'s daughter states, "She won't need home health PT. Once I get her home, she'll get right up." The patient is dependent in amb & lives alone.) This can be used to assist with appropriate placement for the patient and to protect the patient from a potentially unsafe environment.

- To **describe pain.** (Example: Pt. describes pain as "like a knife stabbing right through my Ⓡ thigh.")

▌ Using Information Taken from a Family Member

Information taken from an interview with a patient's family member can be included in the following manner:

 E X A M P L E

Problem: Ⓛstroke c̄ Ⓡhemiparesis & aphasia.
S: (All of the following information was taken from pt.'s daughter. Pt. is unable to verbalize 2° aphasia.) Functional status/activity level: Pt. amb indep PTA. Living environment: Pt. lives c̄ daughter & daughter's husband in a 1-story home c̄ 3 steps c̄ handrail Ⓛascending to enter the home. Home has carpeted & linoleum surfaces s̄ throw rugs. Pt.'s bedroom is ~7 ft. from the bathroom & ~15 ft. from the kitchen or living room. Daughter works full time. Family goals: Pt. must be able to stay alone during the day while daughter works.

Examples of use of a combination of information taken from the patient and a family member follow in corresponding physical therapy and occupational therapy notes regarding the same patient:

 E X A M P L E

Problem: Peripheral neuropathy bilat. LEs; COPD. Hx: Htn, ASHD.
S: Current condition: Pt. c/o SOB ā examination; immediately p̄ examination, indicated that SOB had ↓; 5 min. p̄ exercise, stated SOB had ↓. Medical/surgical hx: Pt's husband stated pt. hx of COPD for 10 yrs. & hx of htn. controlled by medication. Functional status/activity level: Pt. has not amb for the past 2 mo. & has required assist. for transfers 2° SOB & weakness. Husband stated Pt. transferred & amb. s̄ assist. device indep. prior to past 2 mo. Living environment: Husband described a 1-story home; c̄ a ramp to access the entrance. All floor surfaces are linoleum. Farthest distance pt. must amb is ~50 ft. Husband is home full time to care for Pt. Pt. goals: Both stated long term goal of Pt. amb indep, c̄ or s̄ assist. device, & short-term goal of indep. transfers.

Ⓔ X A M P L E

Problem: Peripheral neuropathy bilat. LEs; COPD. Hx: Htn, ASHD.

S: Current condition: Pt. stated she cannot tolerate both PT & OT bid 2° fatigue. Husband states Pt. has needed assist. for dressing LEs, transfers w/c ↔ toilet & has required set-up for a sponge bath with assist. in bathing LEs. Medical/surgical hx: Pt. states 10 yr. hx of COPD. LE weakness began ~2 mo. ago. Functional status/activity level: Husband states Pt. was able to handle all self-care activities until 2 mo. ago. Living environment: Husband is home full time to care for Pt. but states he is having back pain after transferring the Pt. Pt. goals: Both stated functional goal of indep transfers w/c↔toilet, indep in bathing & dressing, & Pt. would like to be able to bathe in the tub or shower.

Writing Interim (Progress) Notes

The *S* portion of the note is optional in an interim note. It is used if there is an update of previous information or if there is relevant new information to convey. Listing information that reflects a temporary mood of discouragement in the patient is not necessary and could confuse those reading the note. Of course, irrelevant information is never appropriate.

Subjective information addressed in previously set goals for the patient should be addressed in the interim note. For example, the patient initially stated that his or her pain prevented the performance of functional activities and rated his or her level of pain using a pain scale. The therapist and patient set a goal for decreasing the patient's pain by three levels on the pain scale in 1 week. Because the pain level and functional activities were addressed in the initial examination and in the goals, the patient's functional level and level of pain should be addressed in the interim note at the end of the week. Although information such as pain level is subjective, it can be a method of showing progress when combined with functional progress.

A patient's subjective **response to treatment interventions**—such as pain following exercise, pain felt with movement, a decrease in pain after treatment, or fatigue after exercise—can be reported in an interim note. This information can be used to document improvement and reinforce objective measurements. For example, if a patient used to feel pain with exercise or a certain movement, such as bending forward or backward, and no longer feels pain, then the patient has improved in pain-free mobility, making him or her more functional in ADLs.

Another type of subjective information that can be addressed in the interim note is information regarding the **patient's compliance and/or other health conditions during the week.** After interviewing the patient, the therapist can document whether the patient is doing prescribed exercises at home and how often. (Example: Pt. states she is performing her exercises in the A.M. & late night time but performs exercises at midday ~50% of the time.) Medical problems, such as cold or flu that could help explain why a patient did not progress during a week or two of therapy, can be documented.

The patient's **functional status/activity level** is still another area that can be addressed in the Subjective section of the note. Unless the therapist sees the patient in the patient's home, she must rely on the patient to convey information about function at home. A patient may appear to be making only minimal progress in therapy on impairments of range of motion or strength (objective measures of the degree of impairment) but may be making large improvements in functional ability at home. Thus, subjective information regarding functional status should be included in interim notes.

Writing Discharge Notes

The completeness of the *S* section of a discharge note varies greatly from facility to facility. In some facilities, the discharge note is similar to an interim note and only updates the patient's status since the most recent interim note was written. In other facilities, the *S* portion of the discharge note more completely summarizes the patient's complaints, living environment, and functional status, comparing the patient's initial status to the discharge status. A discharge note may also list whether the patient believes the goals set were achieved and whether the patient feels ready to function at home. For the purposes of this workbook, the discharge note is to be considered a complete summary of the patient's status upon discharge from therapy, and all of the relevant subjective information regarding the patient should be addressed.

Summary

The *S* portion of the note should include relevant information that will assist the therapist with deciding which tests and measures are needed, setting goals for the patient, planning the treatment interventions, and deciding when to discontinue care. Irrelevant information should not be included, but care needs to be taken to address the patient's current condition, and the functional status and living environment, both at the present time and prior to the onset of the patient's current condition.

The worksheets that follow will give you practice in the skills needed to write the *S* portion of a note. Also included are some exercises in stating the problem. After reviewing Chapter 8, "Stating the Problem," and the material in this chapter, working with the following worksheets, and using the answer sheets to correct the worksheets, you should be able to easily write the problem and subjective portions of a note.

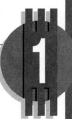

Writing Subjective (S):
Worksheet 1
(Also Included: Stating the Problem)

PART I. Mark the statements that should be placed in the *S* category by placing an *S* on the line before the statement. Also mark the information that belongs in the Problem portion of the note by writing Prob. on the line before the statement.

1. __S-Msw__ Pt. c/o pain (L) wrist.

2. _____ Pt. will demonstrate a normal gait pattern 95% of the time within 3 wks.

3. _____ Flexion in lying reproduces pt.'s worst (R) LE pain.

4. _____ Pulsed US @ 1.5–2.0 W/cm² to (R) upper trapezius for 5 min.

5. _____ <u>Strength:</u> 5/5 throughout all extremities.

6. ___S___ States hx of COPD since 2000.

7. _____ Pt. has good rehab potential.

8. _____ Will be seen by OT 3×/wk. as an O.P.

9. ___S___ States onset of pain was in July 2000.

10. __S-prob__ <u>Hx</u> (from medical record): CA of the colon c̄ colostomy in 2001.

11. _____ <u>AROM:</u> WNL bilat LEs.

12. _____ Pt. has been referred to home health services for further PT & OT.

13. _____ ↑AROM (R) shoulder to WNL within 2 mo.

14. ___S___ Denies pain c̄ cough.

15. _____ Will initiate OT post-op per TKA pathway protocol.

16. __S-prob__ <u>Hx</u> (from medical record): Htn, ASHD, CAD.

17. _____ Pt. was unable to communicate verbally & did not follow commands well; thus, only limited tests & measures performed.

18. _____ Indep in donning/doffing prosthesis within 1 wk.

19. _____ <u>Gait:</u> Independent c̄ crutches 10% PWB (R) LE for 150 ft. × 2.

20. ___S___ C/o pain (L) low back p̄ sitting for ~10 min.

21. _____ Will inquire if pt. can be referred to speech language pathologist.

22. ___S___ States his goal is to return to work ASAP.

PART II. The following is information regarding several patients' diagnoses and chief complaints. This information was taken from the chart or received from the physician's office. Write the information listed in each case into the Problem portion of a note.

1. The patient is an outpatient and the patient's diagnosis received from the physician is "right shoulder bursitis."

   Correct statement: _____

2. The patient had a right-side stroke approximately 1 year ago with residual left hemiparesis. He now comes to you as an outpatient. The patient's present diagnosis from the physician is "left shoulder subluxation." The patient is a 75-year-old white male.

   Correct statement: _____

   _____

   _____

3. The patient is an inpatient with a diagnosis of respiratory failure. She has a history of chronic obstructive pulmonary disease and congestive heart failure. She also has a history of hypertension.

   Correct statement: _____

   _____

PART III. Below you will find the familiar headings discussed for the *S* portion of a note. Each is followed by five blanks (more than are needed for the exercise). Below these headings are statements to be included in the note. Write the number of each statement in the blank following its appropriate heading. The statements you list following each heading should be in the order in which they would logically appear in a note (for instance, 1–5–3 might make more sense than if you were to order them 3–1–5). You may wish to write the note out on a separate piece of paper to assist yourself with this task.

A. <u>Current condition:</u> _____, _____ , _____ , _____ , _____

B. <u>Pt. goals:</u> _____, _____ , _____ , _____ , _____

C. <u>Living environment:</u> _____, _____ , _____ , _____ , _____

D. <u>Functional status/activity level:</u> _____, _____ , _____ , _____ , _____

E. <u>Medical/surgical hx:</u> _____, _____ , _____ , _____ , _____

F. <u>Family health hx:</u> _____, _____ , _____ , _____ , _____

G. <u>Social hx:</u> _____, _____ , _____ , _____ , _____

H. <u>Employment status:</u> _____, _____ , _____ , _____ , _____

1. Pt. c/o Ⓡ shoulder pain "all over the shoulder."

2. States fell at home & landed on a step on Ⓡ shoulder.

3. States lives c̄ husband at home.

4. Describes pain as constant c̄ intensity of 6 (0 = no pain, 10 = worst possible pain).

5. C/o difficulty lifting heavy cooking pots & closing zippers on the back of her clothing.

6. States pain ↓ c̄ rest & is at its worst while Pt. is at work.

7. States she wants to be able to close her zippers & cook s̄ assist. upon completion of therapy.

8. Denies previous shoulder pain/stiffness/inflammation.

9. States was able to fasten all clothing & was completely independent with all cooking activities and activities of daily living prior to her fall at home.

10. States is seeing PT to ↓ Ⓡ shoulder pain & ↑ Ⓡ shoulder motion.

11. Rates overall health as good.

12. States had x-ray & MRI of Ⓡ shoulder c̄ WNL test results.

13. States hx of htn.

14. States family hx of htn.

15. States husband is currently helping her c̄ ADL tasks at home.

16. Pt. is retired.

17. Pt.'s husband is retired & available to help her at all times c̄ ADLs.

18. Pt. has hobby of gardening & is unable to work in the garden at this time 2° Ⓡ shoulder pain.

19. Pt.'s husband does not help pt. in the garden.

20. States drives herself to therapy.

21. States 85 y.o. husband no longer drives.

PART IV. Rewrite the following *S* statements in a more clear, concise, and professional manner. Also, list the heading under which the statement should be placed.

1. States she had a fall in her living room. (Question: What information from the patient would make this statement more informative and useful?)

   a. Heading: _____

   b. Corrected statement: _____

   c. Answer to question: _____

   _____

2. States pain began around 5:00 P.M. a wk. ago Wed.

   a. Heading: _____

   b. Corrected statement: _____

3. States she is kind of sore today in her Ⓡ foot. (Question: What information from the patient would make this statement more informative and useful?)

   a. Heading: _____

   b. Corrected statement: _____

   c. Answer to question: _____

   _____

   _____

4. States she lives in a house. States she has two steps to enter her home. States the steps have a handrail that is on the right when a person is going up the stairs.

   a. Heading: _____

   b. Corrected statement: _____

   _____

5. States the pain goes from her right hand up her right forearm today. The pain is allowing her to type for only 5 minutes at a time.

   a. Heading: _____

   b. Corrected statement: _____

PART V. The following are the notes to yourself that you jotted down while reading the chart and talking with two patients. The first information is from an initial examination; the second information is from a follow-up, interim, or re-examination. (While taking notes for yourself, you did not consult Hospital XYZ's approved abbreviations list.)

From the Chart

58-yr.-old, male
minor ligamentous injury Ⓡ knee

From the Patient

ⓇKnee pain—constant, "burning"—7 on 0–10 scale
↓ pain c̄ rest
↑ pain c̄– walking
No pain bending Ⓡ knee
Never used crutches before
Lives c̄ wife—apartment on 2nd floor—no elevator, 9 steps to enter c̄ handrail on the Ⓛ going ↑
Fell at work—landing on Ⓡ knee 1st
Wants to be able to access apartment independently (short term)
Wants to be able to resume former busy lifestyle, including returning to work as soon as possible (long term)
Occupation—carpenter

1. Write the previous information into the Problem and S portions of a note. Your partial note should be written to be an acceptable part of the patient's medical record at Hospital XYZ (using approved abbreviations).

_____
_____
_____
_____
_____
_____
_____
_____
_____
_____
_____
_____
_____
_____
_____

_____
_____
_____
_____
_____
_____
_____
_____
_____
_____
_____
_____
_____
_____
_____
_____
_____
_____
_____
_____
_____
_____
_____

From the Chart

This is an interim note on an outpatient. You have received no new information from the patient's physician. For your information: the patient's diagnosis is minor ligamentous injury Ⓛ wrist. The patient is a 33-year-old male.

From the Patient

Ⓛ hand & wrist are puffy & feel stiff when the patient tries to move them

Puffiness worse after work

Types at work—up to 8 hrs. a day—MD told him to limit typing to 4 hrs. a day until stops swelling

Pain w/ typing—5 on a 0–10 scale

↓ pain w/ rest

↑ pain w/ grasping or wt. bearing activities Ⓛ UE

Having difficulty adjusting to splint—did not wear it due to rubbing on his thumb

Fell at work yesterday—landed on Ⓛ hand w/ wrist extended so pain has ↑ since last appointment

Went to physician yesterday—x-ray Ⓛ wrist and hand; told by physician that x-ray was negative

Wants to be able to hold a fork w/o pain (new short term)—trouble eating w/ Ⓡ hand—Ⓛ hand dominant

2. Write the previous information into the *S* portion of the note. Your partial note should be written to be an acceptable part of the patient's medical record at Hospital XYZ (using approved abbreviations).

_____

_____

_____

_____

_____

_____

_____

_____

_____

_____

_____

_____

_____

_____

_____

_____

_____

_____

_____

_____

_____

_____

_____

_____

_____

_____

_____

_____

_____

_____

_____

_____

_____

_____

Answers to "Writing Subjective (S): Worksheet 1" are provided in Appendix A.

Writing Subjective (S):
Worksheet 2
(Also Included: Stating the Problem)

2

PART I. In the following you will find the familiar headings discussed for the *S* portion of a note. Each is followed by five blanks (more than are needed for the exercise). Below these headings are statements to be included in the note. Write the number of each in the blank following its appropriate heading. The statements you list following each heading should be in the order in which they would logically appear in a note (for instance, 1–5–3 may make more sense than if you were to order them 3–1–5). You may wish to write the note out on a separate piece of paper to assist yourself with this task.

A. <u>Current condition:</u> _____, _____ , _____ , _____ , _____

B. <u>Living environment:</u> _____, _____ , _____ , _____ , _____

C. <u>Functional status:</u> _____, _____ , _____ , _____ , _____

D. <u>Pt. goals:</u> _____, _____ , _____ , _____ , _____

E. <u>Medical/surgical hx:</u> _____, _____ , _____ , _____ , _____

F. <u>Social hx:</u> _____, _____ , _____ , _____ , _____

G. <u>Employment status:</u> _____, _____ , _____ , _____ , _____

H. <u>Family health hx:</u> _____, _____ , _____ , _____ , _____

1. States fell @ home & fx (L) hip.

2. States needs to be able to amb $\bar{c}$ walker indep. ~15 ft. to return home $\bar{c}$ her husband.

3. States lives $\bar{c}$ husband in her own home

4. Husband is home all day.

5. Describes 3 steps $\bar{c}$ a handrail (L) ascending @ entrance of her home.

6. States hx of "bad heart trouble" but denies pain or difficulty presently. Cannot remember name of heart condition.

7. States used a walker since 1988 when she fx (R) hip.

8. States is hard of hearing.

9. Pt. c/o pain (L) hip $\bar{c}$ standing NWB (L) LE.

10. States would like to return home $\bar{c}$ her husband $\bar{p}$ D/C.

11. Pt. is retired.

12. Family health hx: Both parents died of MI $\bar{p}$ the age of 80 y.o.

PART II. Rewrite the following *S* statements in a more clear, concise, and professional manner. Also, list the heading under which the statement should be placed.

1. Pain is in her right leg down to, but not including, the knee. (Question: What other information regarding the patient's pain would help this statement to be more useful and informative?)

   a. Heading: _____

   b. Corrected statement: _____

   c. Answer to question: _____

   _____

   _____

2. States he depended on his wife to give him a bath before this stroke and he plans to continue to depend on her to give him a bath now.

   a. Heading: _____

   b. Corrected statement: _____

   _____

3. Complains of not being able to put on her clothes by herself.

   a. Heading: _____

   b. Corrected statement: _____

4. Says she never used a walker before this present adm to Hospital XYZ.

   a. Heading: _____

   b. Corrected statement: _____

   _____

PART III. Mark the statements that should be placed in the *S* category by placing an *S* on the line before the statement. Also mark the information that belongs in the Problem portion of the note by writing *Prob* on the line before the statement.

1. _____ Will request an order for OT to assist c̄ dressing.

2. _____ DTRs 2+ throughout LEs except 3+ Ⓡ KJ.

3. _____ Amb training, beginning // bars & progressing to a walker.

4. _____ States was in a car accident & Pt.'s car was hit broadside on the passenger side.

5. _____ Expected Outcome: Indep walker amb 150 ft. ×2 FWB within 2 wks.

6. _____ Examination not complete because Pt. does not follow commands consistently.

7. _____ C/o inability to zip her dresses behind her back.

8. _____ Transfers: Supine↔sit c̄ min. + 1 assist.

9. _____ Proprioception: ↓ noted throughout entire Ⓡ UE.

10. _____ Medical hx: TIA in 1989, ASHD, CHF.

11. _____ C/o pain in "entire" Ⓛ LE c̄ active or passive movement of the knee.

12. _____ AROM Ⓛ knee to 0–90° within 2 wks.

13. _____ BID @ B/S:

14. _____ Pt. will demonstrate knowledge of proper back care & ADL by discussion of ADL c̄ therapist & through 90% correct performance on an obstacle course in back care & ADL.

15. _____ C/o itching in scar Ⓛ wrist ~ 2×/hr.

16. _____ Will request an order for PT for assessment of gross motor functioning.

17. _____ <u>Sensation:</u> Absent to light touch & pin prick throughout L5 distribution on Ⓛ.

18. _____ Pt. will be given written & verbal instruction in home exercise & walking program (attached).

19. _____ States would like to return to his daughter's house until he no longer needs the walker.

PART IV. The following are the notes to yourself that you jotted down while reading the chart and talking with your patient. (While taking notes for yourself, you did not consult Hospital XYZ's approved abbreviations list.)

From the Chart

Diagnosis is contusion left hip.

From the Patient

Ⓛ hip pain when FWB Ⓛ LE—8 on a 0–10 scale.
Total hip replacement Ⓛ 1990—used walker then.
No hip pain sitting or supine.
Apartment with elevator—lives alone—curbs only.
Fell in kitchen on Ⓛ hip in A.M.—able to get up s̄ help—pain throughout day—went to ED late P.M.
Did not use an assistive device before his injury and walked independently.
Did all ADL tasks independently prior to his injury.
Eventually would like to independently perform all ADL tasks s̄ walker.
Currently spends time in a wheelchair rented by the family.
Volunteers at her church—types church bulletin and helps clean.

Write the previous information into the Problem and *S* portions of a note. Your partial note should be written to be an acceptable part of the patient's medical record at Hospital XYZ (using approved abbreviations).

_____

_____

_____

_____

_____

_____

_____

_____

_____

_____

_____

_____

_____

_____

_____

_____

_____

_____

_____

_____

_____

_____

_____

_____

_____

_____

_____

_____

_____

_____

_____

_____

_____

_____

_____

_____

_____

_____

_____

_____

_____

_____

_____

_____

_____

_____

_____

_____

_____

_____

Answers to "Writing Subjective (S): Worksheet 2" are provided in Appendix A.

The SOAP Note: Writing Objective (O)

The *Objective* part of the note is the section in which the results of tests measurements performed and the therapist's objective observations of the patient are recorded. Objective data are the *measurable* or *observable* information used to formulate the plan of care. The testing procedures that produce objective data are *repeatable*. Objective information written in one note can be compared with measurements taken and recorded in the past. It also serves as comparative data in the future, as the patient's progress is monitored and reevaluated.

Categorizing Items into Objective Notes

An item belongs under objective if the item is describing the *systems review* done by the therapist. The purpose of the systems review is to confirm that the patient is appropriate for therapy and to serve as a screening tool for referral to other health professionals. This is usually done during the initial examination of the patient. The systems review includes the following:

- **Cardiovascular/Pulmonary System** information such as heart rate, respiratory rate, blood pressure, or edema. The Cardiovascular/ Pulmonary system is rated as *impaired* or *not impaired* as a whole system, and individual measurements of heart rate, blood pressure, respiratory rate, and a general description of edema are listed.

E X A M P L E

Cardiovascular/Pulmonary System: Impaired. BP: 140/85. HR: 90 bpm. RR: 20. Edema: pitting edema noted bilat. ankles.

- **Integumentary System** information such as integumentary disruption, continuity of skin color, skin pliability, or texture. The Integumentary System as a whole is listed as *impaired* or *not impaired*.

E X A M P L E

Integumentary System: Impaired. Wound noted Ⓡ ant. leg. Skin discolored around area of wound. Skin thin & fragile bilat. LEs.

- **Musculoskeletal System** information such as gross symmetry during standing, sitting, and activities, gross range of motion, gross muscle strength. The patient's height and weight are also recorded with musculoskeletal information. Specific range of motion (ROM) and muscle testing is not reported as part of the systems review. Each subcategory of this section (gross symmetry, gross range of motion, gross muscle strength) is listed as *impaired* or *unimpaired*.

E X A M P L E

Musculoskeletal System: Gross symmetry: impaired in LEs in standing. Gross ROM: unimpaired bilat. LEs. Gross Strength: impaired bilat. LEs, Ⓡ > Ⓛ.

- **Neuromuscular System** information such as gait, locomotion (transfers, bed mobility), balance, and motor function (motor control, motor learning). Specific descriptions of these are not reported in this section of the note. Each individual subcategory (gait, locomotion, balance, motor function) under the Neuromuscular System is reported as *impaired* or *unimpaired*.

E X A M P L E

Neuromuscular System: Gait unimpaired.
Locomotion: transfers impaired. Balance: unimpaired. Motor function: unimpaired.

- **Communication Style or Abilities,** including whether the patient's communication is age-appropriate. Specific communication abilities are reported as impaired or unimpaired.

E X A M P L E

Communication: Age appropriate & unimpaired.

- Information regarding the patient's **Affect,** such as the patient's emotional and behavioral responses. Affective abilities are reported as *impaired* or *unimpaired.*

E X A M P L E

Affect: Emotional/behavioral responses unimpaired.

- Information regarding the patient's **Cognition,** such as whether the patient is oriented to person, place, and time (oriented × 3), or the patient's level of consciousness. Cognitive abilities are reported as *impaired* or *unimpaired,* with specifics mentioned as necessary.

E X A M P L E

Cognition: Level of consciousness unimpaired.
Orientation to person unimpaired; orientation to place & time impaired.

- Information regarding **Learning Barriers** that the patient may have, such as vision, hearing, inability to read, inability to understand what is read, language barriers (needs an interpreter) and any other learning barrier noted by the therapist. It should be noted that the use of glasses and hearing aids is listed in the *History* part of the note under Living Environment: Devices and Equipment. If the patient uses assistive devices that compensate for visual or hearing barriers, these barriers should only be noted if the assistive devices are not available, are not sufficient to compensate for the patient's learning barrier, or if the patient requires additional assistance of some kind.

E X A M P L E

Learning Barriers: Hearing: Pt. understands best when able to see therapist's lips along with use of hearing aid.

- Information regarding the patient's **Learning Style.** This includes reporting *how the patient / client best learns* (e.g., pictures, reading, listening, demonstration, other).

E X A M P L E

Learning Style: Pt. learns best when rationale for exercises is given before demonstration.

- Information regarding the patient's **Education Needs.** This includes reporting areas in which the patient needs more education or information, such as disease process, safety, use of devices and equipment, activities of daily living, exercise program, recovery and healing process and other education needs noted by the therapist. These are reported as a listing of all of the areas in which the patient needs education.

E X A M P L E

Education Needs: Disease process, home exercise program, use of the back in ADLs.

An item also belongs under objective if either of the two following bulleted items apply:

- It is a **result of the therapist's objective tests and measures or observations** (must be measurable and reproducible data; may use database, flow sheets, or charts, to summarize data).

E X A M P L E

O: AROM: WNL throughout UEs & LEs except 120° Ⓛ shoulder flexion noted.

- It is part of the patient's *medical history* taken from the medical record and relevant to the current problem. Note: Only certain facilities include information from the medical record under the Objective section.

E X A M P L E

O: <u>Hx:</u> ASHD, CHF, COPD. S/P fx Ⓛc̄ prosthesis insertion 1 yr.

As mentioned previously, facilities differ widely as to whether information from the medical record becomes part of the therapy note, and, if so, where and how much pertinent information is included. Some therapists believe that if the information is relevant enough to state, it should go with the diagnosis when the patient's problem is stated. Other facilities have the policy that information from the patient's medical record should be included in the Objective section of the note because it is information that the therapist did not obtain from the patient directly (and therefore is not subjective), and the section including the diagnosis is extremely brief. Still other facilities do not include information from the medical record under *O* because it is not a result of direct testing performed by the therapist. On arriving at a facility to practice, students should inquire as to which style of note writing is used. For the purposes of this workbook, you are expected to briefly include information from the medical record after the diagnosis or chief complaint when you initially state the patient's problem.

Abbreviations and Medical Terminology

Appropriate use of abbreviations and medical terminology is expected, as well as correct spelling. The following pages discuss some methods of recording objective data. Use them as a reference. Clarity and conciseness are important.

Organization

Information should be organized, easy to read, and easy to find. Please see the example in the next column.

Categories

To organize objective data better and make it easy to read, objective information is divided into categories

E X A M P L E

Poorly Written

O: Strength is 5/5 throughout UEs. ROM is WNL throughout UEs. Ⓡ toes are warm to touch & coloration is normal. Ⓛ LE AROM is WNL throughout. Ⓡ LE strength & ROM not assessed due to long leg cast. Ⓛ LE strength is 5/5 throughout. Able to manage NWB status Ⓡ LE indep.

Properly Written

O: <u>UEs & LE:</u> Strength & AROM are WNL throughout. Ⓡ LE: Strength & AROM not assessed due to long leg cast. Toes warm to touch & coloration WNL. Able to manage NWB status indep.

or headings. The headings or categories used depend on the patient's deficits and diagnosis.

A category or heading for the Systems Review should always begin the Objective section of a note. Results from tests and measures then follow.

Headings or categories can be based on the *types of tests and measurements performed*. This type of organization is helpful when the patient has deficits in several parts of the body or some type of generalized problem. Examples of categories include the following:

Ambulation
Transfers
Balance
ROM
Strength
Sensation

Headings or categories can also be based on *areas of the body and functional skills*. Use of this type of organization is found when many of the patient's deficits are located in one or two parts of the body. Examples of categories include the following:

Ambulation
ADL
UEs
LEs
Trunk
   Or
Ambulation
ADL
Ⓡ Extremities
Ⓛ Extremities
Trunk

Placement of Objective Data into Categories

Placing objective data into categories depends on the diagnosis and deficits of the individual patient.

E X A M P L E

1. For the physical therapist, a patient with a low back problem may show deficits in the areas of gait, many aspects of the trunk, and the lower extremities, as well as body mechanics during transfers and activities of daily living. The information should be divided into categories that list the information regarding the trunk, lower extremities, and gait separately: gait, ADL, trunk, LEs, UEs. For the occupational therapist, the patient may show deficits in lifting abilities needed in her or his work, body mechanics, and daily self-care activities. The information should be divided into categories listing the deficit areas separately: vocational activities, body mechanics, self-care activities.

2. A patient with a diagnosis of left-sided stroke might show deficits in many aspects regarding the right side of the body including decreased active moment, a change in tone, decreased sensation, changed deep tendon reflexes, decreased coordination, and decreased fine motor abilities. To make the information clearer and the deficits easier to read, the information regarding the right extremities should be separated from that for the left extremities because the left extremities are essentially normal. The trunk is one entity and should not be divided into different categories. Gait deviations and deficits in dressing and grooming exist and should each be described in a separate category. Deficits are found in other functional activities such as transfers and rolling. These functional activities can be listed under the categories of transfers and bed mobility. The categories used by the physical therapist might be gait, transfers, bed mobility, Ⓡextremities, Ⓛextremities, and trunk. The categories used by the occupational therapist might be transfers, bed mobility, dressing, grooming, Ⓡ extremities, and Ⓛextremities.

3. A patient with colon cancer might show many deficits in strength and range of motion. These deficits occur in all of the extremities when the physical therapist assesses the patient. Transfers and ambulation need work. The patient's endurance is low. For the physical therapist, the information might best be divided according to the patient's basic areas of deficit: ambulation, transfers, strength, AROMs, endurance. When the occupational therapist assesses this patient, the patient also shows deficits in UE strength and AROM as well as deficits in endurance, feeding, grooming, and dressing activities. For the occupational therapist, the information might also best be divided according to areas of deficit: feeding, grooming, dressing, UE strength, UE AROMs, endurance.

4. When the therapist assesses a young pediatric patient, the assessment reveals low muscle tone, normal ROM, deficits in strength and stability, a delay in righting reactions, and deficits in mobility. These areas can all be listed under the category of gross motor skills. The child shows appropriate fine motor skills and deficient sensory functioning as well as difficulties in feeding. The therapist chooses to divide the categories into ADL, gross motor, fine motor, and sensory.

Use of categories also varies from one clinical facility to another. Certain facilities require therapists to categorize information on all patients in the same manner despite differences in diagnoses and deficits between patients. (For example, all notes in one facility might have the categories *gait, ADL, strength, ROM, sensation.*) Other facilities give the therapists more freedom to categorize information in the manner they deem most efficient and organized. For the purposes of this workbook, you are expected to choose the most appropriate categories for each patient's specific diagnosis and deficits.

Within the objective portion of a note, the categories can be arranged using a number of different methods. Some clinicians list the functional activities (gait, transfers, ADL) first because they believe that functional activities are the most important. Others believe that the extremities and trunk or tests performed should be listed first because the information on specific impairments (ROM, strength, and so forth), is needed to understand the reasons for the deficits in function. Most of the audiences for SOAP notes (physicians, insurance reviewers, lawyers, case managers, social workers) prefer listing the functional activities first, with the reasons for the deficits in function listed after the functional deficits. For the purposes of this workbook, you are expected to address functional activities before listing the impairments or specific tests performed.

Within any individual category in the objective section of a note, the information is organized in the most logical order possible. Usually one joint at a time is described, and joints are addressed proximally to distally. Information is otherwise grouped as efficiently as possible within this framework.

 X A M P L E

UEs: AROM: WNL bilat. except for 80° ⓡ shoulder flexion & 90° ⓡ elbow flexion. BILAT. STRENGTH: 4–/5 throughout shoulder musculature, 4+/5 biceps, 4/5 triceps, 3/5 in musculature controlling the wrist & fingers. SENSATION: Intact throughout bilat.

Methods of Recording Objective Data

In many facilities, complete sentences are not necessary, but information should be clear enough to get the idea across.

 X A M P L E

Unclear

AROM: ⓛ ankle in cast.

Clear

AROM: ⓛ ankle not examined due to short leg cast ⓛ LE.

At times, using a table gets the information across in the most complete manner.

 X A M P L E

Correct Method

AROM: finger & thumb extension/flexion is as follows:

Digit	MCP	PIP	DIP
1	20-0-45°	10-0-20°	
2	10-0-40°	0-15°	0-2°
3	10-0-40°	0-30°	10-0-5°
4	10-0-38°	0-10°	0-8°
5	20-0-47°	0-5°	0-5°

Sometimes, a standard ROM or muscle testing chart, flow sheet, or some other standardized table can be used (many therapy departments have these available for use). Instead of giving detailed infor-

mation within the note, the therapist can refer to the flow sheet or chart and attach a copy to the note.

 X A M P L E

AROM ⓡ UE: See attached table; limited at shoulder & elbow.

A table or flow sheet should always be dated and signed.

In certain situations in which the patient has very limited or simple problems, the entire SOAP note may be a flow sheet.

Common Mistakes in Recording Objective Data

Some of the most common mistakes in recording objective data are the following:

1. Failure to state the *affected anatomy*
2. Failure to state objective information in *measurable terms*
3. Failure to state the *type* of whatever it is that is being measured or observed

E X A M P L E

Correct

AROM, the type of ROM measured
Shoulder *flexion*, the type of movement measured
Gait deviations, the type of deviations observed
Sliding board w/c ↔ *mat* transfers, the type of transfers observed

If something cannot be stated in measurable terms, the word *appears* instead of *is* should be used.

 X A M P L E

Correct

UE strength not formally tested on this date but appears functional for transfers w/c↔mat.

The term *appears* should be used very cautiously; third-party payers will not provide reimbursement for intervention that "appears" to be needed.

Some Specifics Regarding Recording Objective Data

Using scales with numerical values showing the value of normal—such as 3/5 strength versus fair strength—is suggested to make the job of those reading the notes for third-party payers somewhat easier. Appendix D includes some suggestions regarding recording objective data to maximize the effectiveness of note writing for third-party payers.

Methods for recording objective data along with common tests and measures can be found in *The Guide to Physical Therapist Practice.**

Writing Interim (Progress) Notes

In an interim (progress) note, not every category normally addressed in an initial note is included. Use only the information obtained while re-examining the patient during sessions subsequent to the initial examination and evaluation.

If a patient's status is unchanged and the area addressed is extremely important, it is acceptable to address the area and state that it is unchanged. However, for the sake of the reader, the unchanged status should be described briefly.

E X A M P L E

Correct

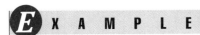

Transfers: Supine↔sit unchanged; still requires mod + 1 assist.

When stating that the patient's status is unchanged, it is important to make sure that all of the tests and measures available have been used. In the previous example, perhaps the amount of assistance needed by the patient is unchanged, but the patient is performing the transfer more quickly (5 minutes to perform the transfer versus the 10 minutes the patient used to require).

E X A M P L E

Correct

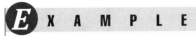

Transfers: Supine↔sit unchanged; still requires mod + 1 assist. but performance of transfer requires 5 min. on this date (vs. 10 min. required on [date]). Transfer is becoming more functional.

The Guide to Physical Therapist Practice.

Data used for comparison purposes can also be included. In the previous example, without the comparative data, the fact that the performance of the transfer required 5 minutes would seem insignificant to the reader. The reader may not take the time to look at a previously written note to obtain the patient's former status, or the previous note may not be available to the reader.

Information addressed in interim notes should include areas addressed in the last set of anticipated goals written. For example, if a goal is set for the patient to be able to "roll supine↔sidelying Ⓡ indep within 1 wk," the patient's rolling status should be addressed under *O* in the next interim note.

As mentioned previously, when writing notes, it is important to know the requirements of both the facility and the third-party payers. In some areas of the country, certain third-party payers require listing both the interventions the patient received and the patient's reaction to the interventions. This can be listed in the *O* part of the note under *Reaction to Interventions.*

E X A M P L E

Correct

Reaction to Rx: Pt. received 30 min. of gait training on this date emphasizing correction of gait deviations & correction of balance deficits. Responded well to verbal cues but could not cont. to correct gait deviations.

Writing Discharge Notes

The completeness of the *O* section of a discharge note varies greatly among practice settings. In some facilities, the discharge note is similar to an interim note and is an update of the patient's status since the last interim note was written. In other facilities, the discharge note is a more complete summary of the patient's condition upon discharge from the facility and, in format and length, is more similar to the initial note. Still other facilities use a format that summarizes the patient's condition upon beginning therapy, the general course of therapy, and the patient's status upon discharge from therapy.

Types of notes can also vary depending on who will be reading the note. For example, a note that is forwarded to a nursing home or home health agency might be a complete summary of the patient's condition, whereas a note that will go the medical records storage when the patient is discontinued may simply update the patient's status since the last interim note was written. The home health or nursing home therapist may receive only the discharge summary from an acute or rehabilitation facility, so a more complete note is needed. For the purposes of this workbook, the discharge note is considered a complete summary of the patient's status upon discharge and course of therapy, and you are to address all areas of objective data measured and remeasured during treatment.

▌Summary

The *O* section of the note is a very important section. It should be included in every type of note, whether it is an initial, interim, or discharge note. The information should be organized under headings, should be written in a clear and concise manner, and should list the results of observations, tests and measures performed by the therapist. The first of the headings listed should always be the Systems Review in the initial note.

The following worksheets give practice at the skills needed to write the *O* part of a note. After reviewing this chapter, working with the following worksheets, and using the answer sheets to correct the worksheets, you should be able to write the Objective portion of a note easily.

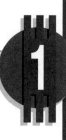

Writing Objective (O):
Worksheet 1

PART I. Mark the statements that should be placed in the *O* category by placing an *O* on the line before the statement. Also mark the *S* items with an *S* and the information that belongs in the Problem portion of the note by writing *Prob.* on the line before the statement.

1. _____ Will receive pulsed US @ 1.5–2.0 W/cm^2 to Ⓡ upper trapezius.

2. _____ <u>Strength:</u> 5/5 throughout all extremities.

3. _____ Pt. has good rehab. potential.

4. _____ Pt. c/o pain Ⓛ ankle.

5. _____ Hip clearing reproduces pain Ⓛ knee.

6. _____ States onset of pain in July 2002.

7. _____ Pt. has been referred to home health services for further Rx.

8. _____ Denies pain c̄ cough.

9. _____ <u>Dx:</u> traumatic brain injury.

10. _____ <u>Transfers:</u> w/c↔mat c̄ sliding board c̄ min + 1 assist.

11. _____ Indep in donning/doffing prosthesis within 1 wk.

12. _____ MUSCULOSKELETAL SYSTEM: Strength impaired Ⓡ UE & LE.

13. _____ C/o pain Ⓛ low back p̄ sitting for ~10 min.

14. _____ Will refer Pt. to speech language pathology.

15. _____ <u>Gait:</u> Indep c̄ crutches 10% PWB Ⓛ LE for 150 ft. × 2.

16. _____ Pt. was difficult to examine due to lack of cooperation as demonstrated by closing his eyes & crossing his arms when given a command.

17. _____ Will initiate OT post-op day 2 per critical pathway.

18. _____ ↑AROM Ⓡ shoulder to WNL within 6 wks.

19. _____ <u>Reaction to Rx:</u> Received training in w/c propulsion & management, transfer training c̄ sliding board w/c↔mat & sit↔supine. Pt. was fatigued p̄ Rx.

20. _____ <u>AROM:</u> WNL bilat LEs.

21. _____ Will be seen by PT as an O.P. beginning c̄ 2×/wk. for 2 wks. & progressing prn.

22. _____ States hx of COPD since 2000.

23. _____ Pt. will be indep in dressing & grooming activities within 2 wks.

PART II. Match each *O* statement with the appropriate heading. More than 1 statement may exist for each heading.

A. <u>Systems Review</u>
B. <u>Amb</u>
C. <u>Transfers</u>
D. <u>Strength</u>
E. <u>ROM</u>
F. <u>Sensation</u>
G. <u>Reaction to Rx</u>

1. _____ UE AROM is WNL except for 0–90° shoulder flexion bilat.

2. _____ ↓ sensation to light touch & pinprick noted in Ⓛ L5 distribution.

3. _____ LE AROM is WNL bilat.

4. _____ Cardiovascular/pulmonary: unimpaired. BP: 120/70. HR: 72. Respiratory Rate: 12. No edema noted.

5. _____ Amb is otherwise WNL.

6. _____ All other UE sensation is WNL.

7. _____ Integumentary System: Unimpaired

8. _____ Strength is 5/5 in all extremities.

9. _____ Pt. was able to correct his gait c̄ verbal cues p̄ Rx.

10. _____ Transfers supine↔sit are indep but too slow to be functional (5 min.).

11. _____ Pt. demonstrates ↓ time spent in stance phase on Ⓛ LE & ↓ step length Ⓡ LE.

12. _____ UE sensation is WNL bilat.

13. _____ Communication: speech impaired. Follows commands well.

14. _____ All other transfers are performed indep & at a functional speed.

PART III. Rewrite the following *O* statements in a more clear, concise, and professional manner. Also, list the heading under which the statement should be placed. (To assist you, an example is given, and some of the problems are in italics in the first few statements.)

Ⓔ X A M P L E

Passive range of motion is limited to 90 *degrees* of flexion in *both* of her hips.

a. Heading: PROM
b. Corrected statement: Hip flexion limited to 90° bilat.

1. The *patient* has 4/4 strength in *both* of her *arms*.

a. Heading: _____

b. Corrected statement: _____

_____

2. Performing a *straight leg raise* on the *left causes* the *patient's* worst back pain.

    a. Heading: _____

    b. Corrected statement: _____

    _____

3. Strength *is* 5/5 in *right* shoulder *muscles*, 4/5 in *right* biceps, 2/5 in *right* triceps, 0/5 in all other *right* arm musculature distal to the elbow. *Left* arm strength is *normal.*

    a. Heading: _____

    b. Corrected statement: _____

    _____

    _____

    _____

4. *Mary ambulates* for *approximately* 150 *feet full weight bearing with* a walker *twice independently.*

    a. Heading: _____

    b. Corrected statement: _____

    _____

5. The patient was short of breath after transferring supine to sit and bed to bedside chair; her respiratory rate increased from 18 breaths per minute before the transfers to 32 breaths per minute immediately after the transfers.

    a. Heading: _____

    b. Corrected statement: _____

    _____

    _____

    _____

6. Left ankle active range of motion is within the normal range.

    a. Heading: _____

    b. Corrected statement: _____

PART IV. The following are the notes to yourself that you jotted down while examining a patient. (While taking notes for yourself, you did not consult Hospital XYZ's approved abbreviations list.)

Cardiovascular OK. Blood Pressure: 110/65, Heart Rate: 75, Resp. Rate: 14.
Integumentary OK.
Musculoskeletal impaired Ⓡ LE.
Neuromuscular impaired gait and locomotion, motor function unimpaired, balance impaired.
Communication age appropriate & unimpaired.
Affect OK.
Cognition unimpaired; oriented—person, place, time.
Learning barriers—none.
Learning style—likes for me to show him prior to him trying to move.
Ed. needs: ambulation with walker and walker safety, transfer safety, protection of cast.
Both UE—strength & AROM—WNL.
Gait—independent—walker—NWB Ⓛ LE—50 ft. twice.

Ⓛ LE—cast—long leg.
Ⓡ LE AROM normal; strength 5/5 throughout.
Transfers—toilet minimal of 1, sit to and from stand independent, supine to and from sit
    independent.
Curb—(1-step c̄ walker)—minimal of 1
Ambulates in & out of door—min + 1—opens & closes door—walker
Ⓛ LE—not examined further

Rewrite each line into an *O* statement. Include the appropriate category before each statement.
(Example: Ⓡ UE: AROMs WNL except 90° Ⓡ shoulder flexion.)

1. Cardiovascular OK. Blood Pressure: 110/65, Heart Rate: 75, Resp. Rate: 14

   O statement: _____

2. Integumentary OK

   O statement: _____

3. Musculoskeletal impaired Ⓡ LE.

   O statement: _____

4. Neuromuscular impaired gait and locomotion, motor function unimpaired, balance
   impaired.

   O statement: _____

5. Communication age appropriate & unimpaired.

   O statement: _____

6. Affect OK

   O statement: _____

7. Cognition unimpaired; oriented—person, place, time

   O statement: _____

8. Learning barriers—none

   O statement: _____

9. Learning style—likes for me to show him prior to him trying to move

   O statement: _____

10. Ed. needs: ambulation with walker and walker safety, transfer safety, protection of cast

   O statement: _____

11. Both UEs—strength & AROM—WNL

   O statement: _____

12. Gait—independent—walker—NWB Ⓛ LE—50 ft. twice

   O statement: _____

13. Ⓛ LE—cast—long leg

   O statement: _____

14. Ⓡ LE AROM normal; strength 5/5 throughout

   O statement: _____

15. Transfers—toilet minimal of 1, sit to and from stand independent, supine to and from sit independent

    O statement: _____

16. Curb—(1-step $\bar{c}$ walker)—minimal of 1

    O statement: _____

17. Ambulates in & out of door—min + 1—opens & closes door—walker

    O statement: _____

18. Ⓛ LE—not assessed further

    O statement: _____

PART V. In the following you will find headings for the *O* portion of a note. Each is followed by blanks (more than are needed for the exercise). Using the statements from Part IV, write the number of each after its appropriate heading. The statements you list after each heading should be in the order in which they would logically appear in a note (for instance, 1–5–3 may make more sense than if you were to order them 3–1–5).

A. Systems Review: _____, _____, _____, _____, _____

B. Amb: _____, _____, _____, _____, _____

C. Transfers: _____, _____, _____, _____, _____

D. UEs & Ⓡ LE: _____, _____, _____, _____, _____

E. Ⓛ LE: _____, _____, _____, _____, _____

PART VI. Using the categories listed previously, use the information to write the *O* portion of a note. (Some of the previous statements may have to be rewritten to combine similar material into a single statement.) Your partial note should be written to be an acceptable part of the patient's medical record at Hospital XYZ (using approved abbreviations).

O: _____

_____

_____

_____

_____

_____

_____

_____

_____

_____

_____

_____

_____

_____

_____

_____

Answers to "Writing Objective (O): Worksheet 1" are provided in Appendix A.

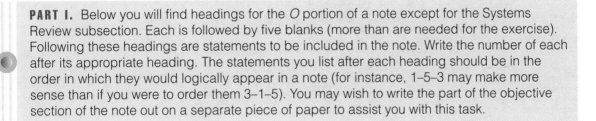

Writing Objective (O):
Worksheet 2

PART I. Below you will find headings for the *O* portion of a note except for the Systems Review subsection. Each is followed by five blanks (more than are needed for the exercise). Following these headings are statements to be included in the note. Write the number of each after its appropriate heading. The statements you list after each heading should be in the order in which they would logically appear in a note (for instance, 1–5–3 may make more sense than if you were to order them 3–1–5). You may wish to write the part of the objective section of the note out on a separate piece of paper to assist you with this task.

A. <u>Gait:</u> ____, ____ , ____ , ____ , ____

B. <u>Transfers:</u> ____, ____ , ____ , ____ , ____

C. <u>(R) extremities:</u> ____, ____ , ____ , ____ , ____

D. <u>(L) extremities:</u> ____, ____ , ____ , ____ , ____

1. All transfers are totally dependent.
2. AROM, strength, & sensation to light touch WNL throughout (R) UE & LE.
3. (L) UE & LE completely flaccid.
4. No active movement noted in (L) extremities.
5. Sensation to light touch intact (L) extremities.
6. Amb not feasible at this time.
7. PROM WNL throughout (L) extremities.

PART II. The following are the notes to yourself that you jotted down during your therapy session while re-examining your patient (for an interim note). (While taking notes for yourself, you did not consult Hospital XYZ's approved abbreviations list.)

Propels w/c himself 15 ft. to mat—difficulty getting close to mat & locking brakes—maximum
    + 1 to place sliding board
Maximum + 1 to remove armrest
W/c↔mat c̄ sliding board & minimum + 1 assist for NWB (R) LE—verbal cues for hand
    placement
Sit↔supine c̄ moderate of 1 to move (R) LE
Hip flex 4/5 (L), 3–/5 (R)
Hip ext 4/5 (L) 3/5 (R)
Knee flex 4/5 (L), 2–/5 (R)
Knee ext 4/5 (L) 3/5 (R)
Ankle 5/5 bilat all movements
Hip abduction bilaterally at least 3/5 bilat; not tested c̄ resistance against gravity
(R) & (L) hip abduction/adduction c̄ 2# × 15 (supine)
(R) & (L) SLR × 15
Knee flex c̄ 2# × 15 (L), 1# × 15 (R)
(L) & (R) terminal knee ext c̄ 2# × 15
Requires frequent rests

Using the categories of your choice, write the above information into the *O* portion of an interim note. Your partial note should be written to be an acceptable part of the patient's medical record at Hospital XYZ.

O: _____

_____

_____

_____

_____

_____

_____

_____

_____

_____

_____

_____

_____

_____

_____

_____

_____

_____

_____

_____

_____

_____

_____

_____

_____

_____

_____

_____

_____

_____

_____

PART III. Rewrite the following *O* statements in a more clear, concise, and professional manner. Also, list the heading under which the statement should be placed.

1. The patient walks 50 feet twice with 50 percent partial weight bearing on her left leg and requires standby assistance from me to compensate for her vision deficits.

   a. Heading: _____

   b. Corrected statement: _____

   _____

2. Examination of the patient's left ankle reveals pitting edema.

   a. Heading: _____

   b. Corrected statement: _____

3. The knee jerk, when tested, is three plus on the right and two plus on the left.

   a. Heading: _____

   b. Corrected statement: _____

4. John used a sliding board to perform his transfer from the wheelchair to the mat and back, requiring my presence to occasionally provide minimal help to stabilize him when he loses his balance.

   a. Heading: _____

   b. Corrected statement: _____

   _____

5. Mary requires two people using maximal assistance to roll her to either side from lying on her back.

   a. Heading: _____

   b. Corrected statement: _____

6. Has no learning problems.

   a. Heading: _____

   b. Corrected statement: _____

   _____

Answers to "Writing Objective (O): Worksheet 2" are provided in Appendix A.

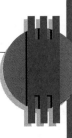
PART I. Indicate which of the following statements are statements that belong in the *Problem, Subjective,* and *Objective* sections of the SOAP note. Mark them by writing *Prob, S,* or *O* on the blank line before the appropriate statement. (Some of the statements do not belong in these sections of the note.)

1. _____ Incision healing well, length 3 in. location immediately prox. to ⓛ thumb-nail.

2. _____ ↑AROM Ⓡ shoulder to WNL within 4 wks. c̄ 3×/wk. Rx.

3. _____ Will instruct Pt. in a home exercise program to improve posture & align-ment (attached).

4. _____ Pt.'s wife states he amb indep s̄ assist. device PTA.

5. _____ DTRs: 2+ throughout.

6. _____ Medical Dx: low back pain.

7. _____ Past experience of PT for low back pain s̄ relief of pain.

8. _____ C/o Ⓡ pain in posterolateral aspects of Ⓡ thigh down to the knee; pain intensity: 8 (0 = no pain, 10 = worst possible pain).

9. _____ Will attempt to perform manual muscle test on another date when Pt. is more rested.

10. _____ X-ray: arthritic spurs L3-5 on the Ⓡ.

11. _____ HR: 75 ā exercise, 95 immediately p̄ exercise, & 75 bpm 3 min. p̄ exercise.

12. _____ Amb s̄ assist. device indep & s̄ deviations

13. _____ Describes onset of pain immed. p̄ lifting a 50 lb. bag of dog food on 01/01/2002.

14. _____ BID: hot pack to low back for 20 min.

15. _____ Pt.'s rehab. potential is guarded.

PART II. Rewrite the following *Problem, Subjective,* and *Objective* statements in a more clear, concise, and professional manner. Also, list the subsection of the notes (*Problem, Subjective,* or *Objective*) and the heading under which the statement should be placed.

1. The patient complains of the left lateral knee pain that comes and goes.

   a. <u>Part of the note:</u> _____ b. <u>Heading:</u> _____

   c. <u>Corrected statement:</u> _____

   _____

2. The patient doesn't have as much sensation in the left L5 dermatome.

   a. <u>Part of the note:</u> _____ b. <u>Heading:</u> _____

   c. <u>Corrected statement:</u> _____

   _____

3. The patient states a doctor "looked in [his] right knee with a scope" on 02/02/2002.

   a. <u>Part of the note:</u> _____ b. <u>Heading:</u> _____

   c. <u>Corrected statement:</u> _____

   _____

4. The patient says he had "surgery where they opened up my skull" in February 2002.

   a. <u>Part of the note:</u> _____ b. <u>Heading:</u> _____

   c. <u>Corrected statement:</u> _____

   _____

5. Right leg passive range of motion is within normal limits throughout.

   a. <u>Part of the note:</u> _____ b. <u>Heading:</u> _____

   c. <u>Corrected statement:</u> _____

   _____

PART III. Here are the notes to yourself that you jotted down while reading the chart and examining your patient. (While taking notes for yourself, you did not consult Hospital XYZ's approved abbreviations list.)

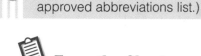

From the Chart

Diagnosis is fractured right femoral neck on 01/12/2002. A right hip prosthesis was inserted on 01/13/2002. Patient is 65 years old. The patient is male. Physician is Dr. Sosome. HgB was 11 this morning. You are seeing the patient on 01/15/2002. You tried to see the patient on 01/14/2002 but patient was dizzy lying in bed and HgB was 7. Patient received blood transfusion on 01/14/2002.

From the Patient

Pain ⓇR hip while standing 8/10, while lying (before ambulation) 4/10

No PT or OT before—no walker or cane before this admission—no tub chair or portable commode currently available at home—no other assistive devices used for dressing, bathing, ambulating

Fell at home and hit Ⓡ hip on side of bathtub

Lives alone—senior apartment building—elevator—curbs only

Apartment bathroom has a bathtub with a shower and shower curtain

Retired this year—was a teacher—still volunteers at elementary school 3 days per week, reading with small children

For recreation, patient watches her grandchildren and plays cards with friends. Watches toddler-aged grandchildren once per week and plays cards with friends 2 nights per week

Would like to return to her apartment after discharge

(For PTs:) Would like to eventually ambulate independently s̄ device once again

(For OTs:) Would like to able to manage grooming and dressing by herself; would "settle" for Meals on Wheels

Walks approximately 2 miles 3 times per week
Does not drink alcohol and does not smoke

Systems Review

Blood pressure was 140/80.
Initially pulse rate was 80.
Respiratory rate was 12.
Neuromuscular system: gait impaired, locomotion impaired, balance impaired in standing and during ambulation, motor function unimpaired.
Integumentary system: impaired at surgery site; otherwise WNL.
Musculoskeletal system: gross strength impaired on the right as is the range of motion.
Communication is unimpaired.
Affect: the patient's emotional/behavioral responses are unimpaired.
Cognition: oriented to person, place, and time; unimpaired.
Learning barriers: patient wears glasses and cannot read without them—therefore, will need them for the home exercise program.
Learning style—likes to be shown by the therapist and then tries to imitate therapist's actions—visual learner.
Education needs—needs to learn how to use a walker on level surfaces and on curbs, needs to learn transfers, needs to learn to check for proper healing of wound, needs a home exercise program.

PT Examination Performed

UEs—ROMs WNL except –5 degrees of right elbow extension.
UEs—strength 4+/5 throughout (group muscle test).
ROMs in left leg WNL.
Right LE—ROMs limited secondary to post-op restrictions to 90 degrees hip flexion, full active hip abduction, zero degrees hip medial and lateral rotation, 0 degrees adduction.
Left LE—strength 4+/5 throughout (group muscle tests).
Right LE—strength at least 3/5 throughout—not further examined due to recent surgery.
Transfers   w/c to and from bed c̄ moderate of 1 person
         Sit to and from stand with minimal of 1 person
         Supine to and from sit with moderate of 1 person
Ambulated—parallel bars minimal of 1 approximately 20 feet once 50% PWB right LE—felt dizzy and nauseated—no further examination or interventions performed this date—nurses notified.
BP: 145/90 immediately after ambulation, 135/80 3 min. after ambulation.
Pulse 105 immediately after ambulation, 82 3 min. after ambulation.
Breathing rate: 18 immediately after ambulation; 12 3 min. after ambulation.

OT Examination Performed

UE strength 4+/5 throughout (group muscle test).
UE—AROM WNL except –5 degrees right elbow extension.
Fine motor skills within normal limits.
Transfers supine to and from sit with moderate assistance of 1.
Transfers wheelchair to and from bed with moderate assistance of 1.
Patient initially seen bedside for assessment of grooming and dressing skills.
Currently has IV infusing in left forearm.
Patient able to bathe UE and trunk but needs minimal assistance of 1 for both LEs and needs setup for sponge bath.
Able to groom his hair independently.
Able to care for his teeth independently.
Wears contact lenses; able to care for lenses by himself from a wheelchair.
Dressing not assessed this date due to high pain level and low patient endurance.

Write the previous information into the *Problem, Subjective,* and *Objective* portions of either a physical therapy note or an occupational therapy note. Your partial note should be written to be an acceptable part of the patient's medical record at Hospital XYZ.

_____

_____

_____

_____

_____

_____

_____

_____

_____

_____

_____

_____

_____

_____

_____

_____

_____

_____

_____

_____

_____

_____

_____

_____

_____

_____

_____

_____

_____

_____

Answers to Review Worksheet: Stating the Problem, S, and O can be found in Appendix A.

Documenting the Evaluation (A)

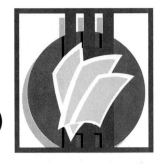

After a health-care professional performs an examination, the next step is the process of making clinical decisions. This process includes determining a patient's diagnosis and prognosis. Part III of Writing SOAP Notes, third edition, covers the Diagnosis (Chapter 11) and Prognosis (Chapter 12) parts of the note.

The Patient/Client Management note has two sections called *Diagnosis* and *Prognosis.* In the SOAP note, the Diagnosis and Prognosis parts of the note are listed in a section called the *Assessment.* This section includes the process of evaluation. In some facilities, the expected outcomes and anticipated goals are listed in the Assessment part of the note.

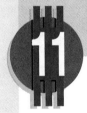

11 Writing the Diagnosis

After the therapist completes the examination, the process of evaluation begins. The therapist looks at the patient's functional deficits and impairments, and places them in a diagnostic category, or practice pattern, as listed in *The Guide to Physical Therapist Practice.** The therapist also looks at more specific movement dysfunction categories that fit under the practice pattern and may more specifically describe the patient's functional deficits and impairments by describing the patient's condition using one or more of those categories. This is the portion of managing the patient/client that only therapists perform. As

The Guide to Physical Therapist Practice.

part of a discussion of the therapy diagnosis, several kinds of information may be addressed. Each category of information is briefly described in the following text and includes a discussion of the therapy diagnosis and the medical diagnosis.

Differences between a Therapy Diagnosis and a Medical Diagnosis

A therapy diagnosis describes the impact functional deficits or impairments have on the person's ability to function in his or her environment. These are the functional deficits or impairments toward which the therapists direct therapy interventions. A medical diagnosis uses categories to describe medical signs and symptoms and directs medical interventions toward these signs and symptoms.

As the therapist performs an evaluation, if the examination reveals findings that do not fall within the scope of therapy practice, the therapist refers the patient to other practitioners who are educated to intervene appropriately with those findings. Physicians refer to other practitioners, including therapists, to intervene more specifically with patient problems that fall within the scope of therapy practice.

Drawing Correlations and Justifying Decisions

The Diagnosis subsection note provides an opportunity for the therapist to describe the connections between the examination findings that would not necessarily be obvious to all parties who read patient care notes. It should describe how impairments relate to the functional deficits and how these functional deficits keep the patient from functioning in his or her specific environment.

> **E X A M P L E**
>
> ↓ Ⓡ shoulder AROM is preventing Pt. from reaching into overhead cabinets. This prevents Pt. from taking care of herself in her home. Ⓡ knee ↓ AROM is preventing Pt. from becoming indep. in amb. c̄ walker & in coming sit ↔ stand. Pt. cannot return to her prior status of living alone in the community until she is able to amb. s̄ walker & transfer sit ↔ indep.

The diagnosis section of the note can include a brief summary of the examination findings that led the therapist to place the patient in a specific practice pattern or movement dysfunction diagnosis.

> **E X A M P L E**
>
> Pt. has hx of diabetes & prior Ⓛ foot ulcers, ↓ ROM & strength Ⓛ foot & ankle, shoes s̄ orthotics that do not fit, ↓ sensation Ⓛ foot, placing Pt.'s condition in Integumentary Pattern A: Primary Prevention/Risk Reduction for Integumentary Disorders.

Secondary Practice Patterns/ Movement Dysfunctions

At times, the patient may have multiple functional deficits or impairments that could place the patient in more than one practice pattern or diagnostic category. In these cases, it is appropriate to list the secondary practice patterns or diagnostic category(s) and explain the rationale for the listing of practice patterns as primary or secondary. It is also appropriate to discuss the progression of a patient from one diagnostic pattern to another, as needed.

> **E X A M P L E**
>
> Primary diagnostic category on this date is Cardiovascular/Pulmonary Pattern C: Impaired Ventilation, Respiration/Gas Exchange, and Aerobic Capacity/Endurance Associated with Airway Clearance Dysfunction due to the medical dx of Ⓡ lower lobe pneumonia. Secondary dx is Musculoskeletal Pattern G: Impaired Joint Mobility, Muscle Performance and Range of Motion Associated with Fx that correlates with the medical dx of fx Ⓡ femoral neck. As pneumonia clears, Musculoskeletal Pattern G will become the 1° practice pattern.

Inconsistencies

In the Diagnosis portion of the note, the therapist has the opportunity to pinpoint inconsistencies between examination findings.

> **E X A M P L E**
>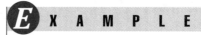
>
> Although patient states entire Ⓛ LE is so painful that it inhibits normal walking, patient amb. over 500 ft. on treadmill FWB s̄ assist. device s̄ gait deviations.

Further Testing Needed

Testing procedures that would be helpful but could not be completed during the initial therapy session can be listed.

> **E X A M P L E**
>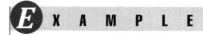
>
> Further testing of sensation & proprioception is needed.

Referral to Another Practitioner

Reasons for referral to another practitioner may be discussed in this section.

 E X A M P L E

Examination revealed increased size of lymph nodes inferior to the Ⓛ clavicle. Examination and evaluation by a physician is indicated. Pt. referred to her primary care physician for medical examination and evaluation of Ⓛ subclavicular area.

Summary

The Diagnosis portion of the Patient/Client Management Note or the SOAP note is extremely important. It places the patient's functional deficits and impairments into a practice pattern and may identify a more specific movement dysfunction category. It may summarize or correlate findings that led the therapist to place the patient's condition into a practice pattern or movement dysfunction category. It may address inconsistencies that may be noted during a patient examination. The Diagnosis part of the note, as a whole, requires much professional judgment. Experience will enable the new practitioner to write this section of the note more easily and without assistance.

The worksheets that follow Chapter 12 will give you practice writing the Diagnosis and Prognosis notes. After reviewing the previous information, completing all of the worksheets, and comparing your work to the answer sheets, you should be able to write the Diagnosis portion of the note with assistance in identifying the specific practice pattern and making connections between examination results and the patient's ability to function in his or her environment.

CHAPTER

Writing the Prognosis

After the therapist completes the examination and determines a therapy diagnosis, the therapist then determines a prognosis. The therapist looks at the severity of the patient's functional deficits and impairments, the patient goals, and living environment, and predicts a level of improvement in function and the amount of time needed to reach the level. This is part of the patient/client management process that only therapists perform. As part of a discussion of the prognosis, several kinds of information may be addressed. Each category of information is briefly described in the following text.

Factors Influencing the Prognosis

A discussion of factors influencing the prognosis such as living environment, patient's condition prior to the onset of the current therapy diagnosis, and current illnesses or medical conditions may be included.

 E X A M P L E

With current medical dx of CA, Pt.'s poor functioning in the home PTA, and the stairs the Pt. must amb. daily @ home, return to home alone is not a safe alternative.

Justification for the Goals Set, the Treatment Plan, and/or Clarification of the Problem

The Prognosis part of a note might include a statement justifying unusual goals. For example, a therapist might get a patient with a diagnosis of stroke who has the potential to transfer independently. However, the patient's wife has been helping to

transfer him for years. Both he and his wife are satisfied with the situation and do not want to change the way they have been living. You might then set your goal: "Pt. will perform all transfers c̄ min assist. from his wife within 1 mo." You would comment: "Due to Pt.'s previous functional level of requiring assist. for transfers from his wife, & Pt. & wife's desire to return to the previous functional level only, a goal of indep transfers is not realistic."

Justification for Further Therapy

The Prognosis portion of a note could also include justification for further therapy for a patient who initially appears relatively independent with one functional activity.

 E X A M P L E

Although amb is indep, Pt.'s progress toward indep transfers is slower. Pt. cont. to need assist. & will benefit from further therapy to work toward indep transfers.

Discussion of Patient's Progress in Therapy

A discussion of the patient's progress in therapy could include further explanation of the patient's failure to progress as quickly as the goals predicted. It could also explain why a patient suddenly regresses or progresses more quickly than anticipated.

 E X A M P L E

Pt. has become more dependent in transfers during the past 2 wks. 2° inactivity associated with patient's recent medical dx of pneumonia.

Future Services Needed

Community services that would be helpful to the patient or may be helpful to the patient in the future can be discussed.

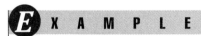

Pt. would benefit from home health physical therapy p̄ D/C from the hospital.

❚ Summary

The Diagnosis portion of the Patient/Client Management Note or the SOAP Note is an important part of the note that documents the therapist's professional opinion about the level of improvement that may be attained.

The worksheets that follow this chapter will give you practice writing the Diagnosis and Prognosis. After reviewing the previous information, completing all of the worksheets, and comparing your work to the answer sheets, you should be able to write the Prognosis portion of the note with assistance in identifying the level of improvement that the patient may reach and time frames that may be required to reach that level.

Writing the Diagnosis and Prognosis:
Worksheet 1

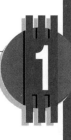

1. _____ <u>Strength:</u> Grossly 2/5 throughout all extremities.

2. _____ <u>Musculoskeletal System:</u> Gross strength impaired all extremities.

3. _____ C/o pain Ⓡ knee of intensity of 6 on a 0–10 scale (0 = no pain; 10 = worst possible pain).

4. _____ States gradual onset of pain in [month, year].

5. _____ Pt. states healing process of residual limb was slowed by infection; took 5 months to heal.

6. _____ Indep. in donning/doffing prosthesis within 1 wk.

7. _____ Will discuss referral to a dietitian c̄ Pt.'s physician.

8. _____ ↑AROM Ⓡ shoulder to WNL within 6 wks. to enable Pt. to reach items in her overhead cabinets.

9. _____ Pt.'s weight will cause progress in PT to be somewhat slow; anticipate a course of therapy for 8 weeks 3×/wk. as an OP.

10. _____ <u>Medical dx:</u> B/K amputation Ⓡ LE.

11. _____ Pt. has been confined to a w/c while residual limb healing occurred.

12. _____ <u>Pt. goals:</u> To return home s̄ assist. p̄ 2 wks. of Rx.

13. _____ Pt. is young and had a high level of function prior to amputation; therefore, rehab. prognosis is good.

14. _____ <u>PROM:</u> WNL bilat. LEs.

15. _____ Learning barriers: very hard of hearing; does not wear hearing aid.

16. _____ Pulsed US underwater at 1.5–2.0 W/cm^2 to Ⓡ wrist.

17. _____ Medical hx of TIA in 2000, ASHD, CHF.

18. _____ Rehab. prognosis guarded. Pt.'s level of function PTA was low. Return to this level will be difficult c̄ further deconditioning 2° prolonged bedrest.

19. _____ Practice pattern Musculoskeletal J: Impaired Motor Function, Muscle Performance, ROM, Gait, Locomotion, & Balance Associated c̄ Amputation.

20. _____ Pt. will progress much more quickly p̄ Pt. is allowed to be FWB Ⓛ LE.

21. _____ States hx of COPD since 2001.

22. _____ Hip clearing reproduces pain Ⓛ knee.

PART II. Determine which of the following statements should be placed in the Diagnosis part of the note and which should be placed in the Prognosis part of the note. Mark the statements that should be placed in the Diagnosis part of the note by writing *Diag.* on the line before the statement. Mark the statements that should be placed in the Prognosis part of the note by writing *Prog.* on the line before the statement.

1. _____ Pt.'s c/o fall outside of the practice area of physical therapy. Contacted Pt.'s physician and Pt. was sent to the Emergency Room for immediate attention.

2. _____ Rehab. potential is good; will progress quickly to independence.

3. _____ Pt. will need Home Health PT p̄ D/C from the hospital to cont. toward indep. on steps Pt. must amb. @ home.

4. _____ ↓ Ⓡ ankle AROM is causing Pt.'s gait deviations. Gait deviations are preventing Pt. from returning to indep. amb. in the community s̄ assist. device. Pt. is required to be indep. s̄ assist. device to return to work.

5. _____ Prognosis is good for complete rehab; however, progress will be slowed by Pt.'s medical dx of COPD.

PART III. Rewrite the following statements into the Diagnosis and Prognosis parts of the note.

1. The results of the examination reveal that the patient's condition falls into two categories: Musculoskeletal pattern G for the patient's fx Ⓛ radius and ulna and Neuromuscular pattern D for the stroke with left-sided hemiplegia. Musculoskeletal Pattern G = Impaired Joint Mobility, Muscle Performance, & ROM Associated With Fracture. Neuromuscular Pattern D = Impaired Motor Function & Sensory Integrity Associated With Nonprogressive Disorders of the Central Nervous System—Acquired in Adolescence or Adulthood. You believe that the primary practice pattern is Neuromuscular Pattern D because the deficits involved are greater, such as significant gait deviations, need to use an assistive device in gait with assistance, and inability to use the left arm in a functional manner. You believe the patient has good rehabilitation potential. She is relatively young, motivated, cooperative, and cognitively sound. The inability to use her left arm in a functional manner is affecting her ability to perform ADLs, and her gait deviations and need for assistance in ambulating with an assistive device prevent her from functioning at home independently and from doing her work as a cashier outside of the home.

_____

_____

_____

_____

_____

_____

_____

_____

_____

_____

_____

_____

2. After performing an examination, you determine that your patient falls into Musculo-skeletal Pattern J: Impaired Joint Mobility, Motor Function, Muscle Performance, and Range of Motion Associated With Amputation. The patient has had an amputation below the knee on the right. You believe the patient's rehabilitation potential is fair because the patient has a medical diagnosis of Alzheimer's Disease. The patient lives on an Alzheimer's Unit in a nursing home. The patient follows simple commands and you believe the patient could become functional at transferring bed↔w/c with minimal assistance and verbal cues. This would assist the nursing home staff in caring for the patient (decrease risk to his caretakers) and would maximize his activity level and quality of life and would further prevent any pulmonary and integumentary problems. The patient's decreased function in transfers is impairing his ability to participate in activities in the nursing home and is placing the health of the nursing home staff at risk.

Answers to "Writing Diagnosis and Prognosis: Worksheet 1" are provided in Appendix A.

Writing the Diagnosis and Prognosis:

Worireet 2

PART I. Mark the statements that should be placed in the Diagnosis part of the note by writing *Diag.* on the line before the statement. Mark the statements that should be placed in the Prognosis part of the note by writing *Prog.* on the line before the statement. Some statements will belong in neither the Diagnosis nor Prognosis part of the note. Also mark the Problem statements with *Prob.*, Subjective statements with an *S*, and the Objective statements by writing *O* on the blank line before the statement.

1. _____ States was in a car accident & Pt. was thrown from car.

2. _____ Indep. walker amb. 150 ft. × 2 FWB within 2 wks. to allow Pt. to amb. from her car into her house.

3. _____ <u>Cognition:</u> Pt. is not oriented to date, place or task & does not follow instructions consistently.

4. _____ <u>Transfers:</u> Supine↔sit c̄ min. + 1 assist.

5. _____ <u>Proprioception:</u> ↓ noted throughout entire Ⓡ LE.

6. _____ Will see BID @ B/S

7. _____ Musculoskeletal practice pattern H: Impaired Joint Mobility, Motor Function, Muscle Performance, & ROM Associated c̄ Joint Arthroplasty.

8. _____ C/o inability to dress indep.

9. _____ Hx of osteoarthritis since 200X.

10. _____ DTRs 2+ throughout LEs except 3+ Ⓡ KJ noted.

11. _____ ↓ ROM & strength Ⓡ LE are associated c̄ Pt.'s gait deviations & dependence in amb. Gait deviations & dependence in amb. prevent Pt. from functioning indep. @ home.

12. _____ Learning style: Pt. prefers to watch a demonstration ā attempting a new activity; visual learner.

13. _____ C/o pain in "entire" Ⓛ LE c̄ active or passive movement of Ⓛ knee.

14. _____ Pt. has excellent rehab. potential.

15. _____ Pt. will need 1–2 home health care visits to teach Pt. to amb. steps @ home.

16. _____ <u>Sensation:</u> Absent to light touch & pinprick throughout C5 distribution.

17. _____ Gross strength impaired Ⓛ LE.

18. _____ 2° practice pattern is Integumentary Pattern C: Impaired Integumentary Integrity Associated With Partial-Thickness Skin Involvement & Scar Formation.

19. _____ Pt. has partial-thickness open wound plantar surface of Ⓛ foot on 1st MP joint 1 cm × .8 cm in size.

20. _____ Amb. will progress quickly once Ⓛ foot is healed.

PART II. Determine which of the following statements should be placed in the Diagnosis part of the note and which should be placed in the Prognosis part of the note. Mark the statements that should be placed in the Diagnosis part of the note by writing *Diag.* on the line before the statement. Mark the statements that should be placed in the Prognosis part of the note by writing *Prog.* on the line before the statement.

1. _____ Pt.'s rehab. potential is poor. Pt. did not cooperate with initial examination 2° cognitive confusion.

2. _____ Will refer to social services to assist. Pt.'s daughter c̄ appropriate ways to deal c̄ the Pt.'s obstinate behavior.

3. _____ Cardiovascular/Pulmonary Practice Pattern: Primary Prevention/Risk Reduction for Cardiovascular/Pulmonary Disorders.

4. _____ Pt. could benefit from PT in the nursing home to which she is transferring. Pt. needs work on indep. & safe amb.

5. _____ ↑ muscle spasm in lumbar paraspinal musculature, ↓ trunk ROM & ↓ ability to tolerate sitting is causing Pt. to ↓ hrs. @ work.

PART III. Rewrite the following statements into the Diagnosis and Prognosis parts of the note.

1. The results of the examination reveal that the patient's condition falls into the Musculoskeletal practice pattern G for the patient's fx Ⓡ radius and ulna. Musculoskeletal Pattern G = Impaired Joint Mobility, Muscle Performance, & ROM Associated with Fracture. The patient's decreased ROM and strength in the Ⓡ wrist are causing the patient to have difficulty c̄ ADLs such as eating & writing. The patient's work involves typing for more than 50% of the time & she is currently unable to type s̄ pain. You believe that the patient has good rehabilitation potential. You believe the patient should progress well with PT.

_____

_____

_____

_____

_____

_____

_____

_____

_____

_____

_____

_____

_____

_____

_____

_____

_____

2. The patient's Ⓡ extremity strength, motor planning, and mobility impairments will prevent the patient from returning home alone. The patient will need to regain independent ambulation and ADLs to return home. The results of the examination reveal that the patient falls into the Neuromuscular Practice Pattern D: Impaired Motor Function & Sensory Integrity Associated c̄ Nonprogressive Disorders of the CNS—Acquired in Adolescence or Adulthood. The patient's rehabilitation potential is fair. The patient may need prolonged time to regain movement of Ⓛ extremities & overall mobility because of her advanced age.

_____
_____
_____
_____
_____
_____
_____
_____
_____
_____
_____
_____
_____
_____
_____
_____
_____
_____
_____
_____
_____
_____
_____
_____
_____
_____
_____
_____

Answers to "Writing Diagnosis and Prognosis: Worksheet 2" are provided in Appendix A.

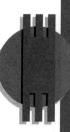

Review Worksheet:

History, Systems Review, Tests & Measures, Diagnosis, Prognosis

Problem, S, O, A

PART I. Begin by turning to the corresponding answer sheets at the end of these instructions so that you can write your partial Patient/Client Management and SOAP notes directly on the answer sheet.

The following are notes to yourself that you jotted down while reading the chart, interviewing, and performing a systems review and tests and measures on your patient. (While taking notes for yourself, you did not consult Hospital XYZ's approved abbreviations list nor were you particularly careful in your notation style.)

1. Write the information into the *History, Systems Review, and Tests and Measures* parts of a Patient/Client Management Note. (Further instructions will be provided to help you write the *Diagnosis and Prognosis* parts of the note.) Your partial note should be written to be an acceptable part of the patient's medical record at Hospital XYZ.

2. Write the information into the *Problem, S, O, and A* parts of a SOAP Note. Your partial note should be written to be an acceptable part of the patient's medical record at Hospital XYZ

 From the Chart

The medical diagnosis is degenerative joint disease Ⓡ hip—total hip replacement performed on [date]
History of htn.
Takes [antihypertensive medication]
65 y.o. male
Dr. Sienn
One prior hospitalization—for Left total hip replacement 01/10/2000

From the Interview

Ⓡ hip pain—area of sutures—intensity of 7 when moving—intensity of 3 when sitting
(0 = no pain, 10 = worst possible pain)—intensity of 2 when lying still
Prior to adm.—intensity of pain was 9 or 10 and pain was constant
1 step at home to get into the house—railing on Ⓡ going up
Owns a 3-in-1 commode, a walker, and a cane
Previous left total hip replacement 01/10/2000
Immediately prior to admission—no assistive device
Lives w/ wife—in his own home
Retired—hobby is gardening
Plans to return home with his wife after D/C
Eventually wants to return to gardening and yard work activities
Does not recall precautions for patients with total hip replacements
Does volunteer ushering at church—also does gardening outside of the church

Right handed dominant
Does not smoke; only occasionally drinks ETOH
Tried to walk for exercise daily—only ambulated one block prior to admission; two years ago
    ambulated a mile or more
Rates general health as good
Has had no major life changes in the past year
Pt.'s father died of MI at age 78
Pt.'s mother died of breast cancer at age 72
Pt. has no siblings

Systems Review

Cardiovascular/pulmonary: not impaired
HR: 80
Resp. rate: 14
BP: 130/85
Edema: none noted
Integumentary: impaired
Disruption: staples (R) hip
Continuity of skin color: WNL
Skin texture: not tested this date
Musculoskeletal:
Gross symmetry: not impaired
Gross ROM: impaired (R) hip and knee
Gross Strength: impaired (R) hip and knee
Height: 6 ft. 0 in.
Weight: 185 pounds
Neuromuscular system:
Gait: impaired
Locomotion: impaired transfers and bed mobility
Balance: impaired in standing—uses walker; not impaired in sitting
Motor function: not impaired
Communication: not impaired
Cognition: oriented × 3; not impaired
Learning barriers: wears glasses—cannot read w/o glasses
Education needs: home exercise program, precautions for patients with total hip replace-
    ment, progression of recovery process, use of walker, ADLs, including transfers
Learning style: demonstration, then trying an activity

From the Tests & Measures Performed

Sit to/from stand w/ moderate of 1
Supine to and from sit with minimal of 1
W/c to/from mat pivot with moderate of 1
Toilet transfers not tested this date
UE AROM WNL
UE strength 4+/5 throughout bilaterally (group muscle test)
(L) LE strength 4/5 throughout (individual muscle testing performed)
(L) LE AROM WNL throughout
Right LE—strength grossly 1/5 in hip and knee musculature—ankle dorsiflexion 4+/5—
    ankle plantar flexion at least 2/5 but not tested further because of the restricted weight
    bearing status
Right LE—AROM—WNL ankle—PROM 0–20° hip flexion, 0–10° hip abduction, 0° hip exten-
    sion—adduction of hip, medial and lateral rotation not tested because of hip precautions
    and recent surgery—knee: 0–70°
Incision—(R) hip—10 cm long—staples intact—over greater trochanter right—healing well
Stood bedside with walker moderate of 1 for 1 minute × 2—10% PWB right LE

Writing Diagnosis

Your opinion is that independent ambulation with a walker is necessary for the patient to go home with a walker. Impairments of decreased ROM and strength right LE are preventing patient from independently ambulating on this date.

The patient fits into Practice Pattern Musculoskeletal H: Impaired Joint Mobility, Motor Function, Muscle Performance & ROM Associated With Joint Arthroplasty.

Prognosis

The patient has good rehabilitation potential. His level of function was good prior to admission and he has a great desire to return to a healthy, active lifestyle in the community. The patient should be able to return to home with his wife independent in ambulation and a home exercise program to continue to increase right LE strength and ROM after 3–4 days of therapy BID.

PART II. Use this answer sheet to write the *History, Systems Review, Tests and Measures, Diagnosis and Prognosis* parts of a Patient/Client Management Note.

_____

_____

_____

_____

_____

_____

_____

_____

_____

_____

_____

_____

_____

_____

_____

_____

_____

_____

_____

_____

_____

_____

_____

_____

_____

_____

_____

_____

_____

_____

_____

_____

_____

_____

_____

PART III. Use this answer sheet to write the *Problem, S, O and A* parts of a SOAP Note.

Answers to "Review Worksheet: History, Systems Review, Tests & Measures, Diagnosis, Prognosis; Problem, S, O, A" are provided in Appendix A.

Documenting the Plan of Care (P)

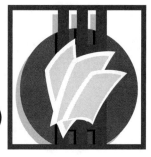

After a health-care professional performs the examination and evaluation process, the next step is determining a plan of care. This process includes writing expected outcomes and anticipated goals for the patient and choosing interventions to help the patient achieve the expected outcomes and anticipated goals. Part IV of Writing SOAP Notes, third edition, covers the Expected Outcomes (Chapter 13), Anticipated Goals (Chapter 14), and Intervention Plan (Chapter 15) parts of the note.

The Patient/Client Management Note has three sections of the plan of care called *Expected Outcomes, Anticipated Goals,* and *Intervention Plan.* In the SOAP Note, the Expected Outcomes, Anticipated Goals, and Intervention Plan parts of the note are listed in a section called the Plan of Care (P).

Writing Expected Outcomes (Long-Term Goals)

The Plan of Care part of the note is the same for both the Patient/Client Management Note and the SOAP Note. It contains a section of Expected Outcomes, a section of Anticipated Goals, an Intervention Plan, and Discharge Plans. Many facilities provide a place for the patient or family member to sign in proof of informed consent.

Expected outcomes describe the final product to be achieved by therapy. After completing the examination and evaluation, including a therapy diagnosis and prognosis, the therapist sets Expected Outcomes. These outcomes are listed in terms of func-

tion. This chapter addresses the process of writing Expected Outcomes.

Reasons for Writing Expected Outcomes

Expected outcomes are written (1) to help you plan interventions to meet the specific needs and problems of the patient, (2) to set priorities between interventions and measure the effectiveness of the interventions, (3) to assist with monitoring cost

133

effectiveness (for purposes of third-party payment), and (4) to communicate the therapy goals for the patient to other health-care professionals.

The Structure of Outcomes and Goals

Before writing Expected Outcomes specifically, it is necessary to know the ABCs of writing objectives. Like an educational objective, a good outcome or goal for patient care contains the following four elements:

A. Audience (who will exhibit the skill)
B. Behavior (what the person will do)
C. Condition (what circumstances—the position, the equipment, and so forth—must be provided or be available for the person to perform the behavior)
D. Degree (how well will the behavior be done—number of feet, number of times performed, amount of assistance needed [i.e., the amount of improvement you want to see specifically])

Audience

Almost always, the patient is the audience. However, it can be a family member or the patient with a family member, as in "Pt. c̄ his wife will be indep. in stairs & curbs s̄ assist. device." Often the audience is implied in writing outcomes or goals, and it is not necessary to say "Pt. will demonstrate..." or Pt. will be..."

The audience is *never* the therapist. Outcomes are patient-oriented, not therapist-oriented.

Behavior

Behavior is always a verb, often followed by the object of the behavior. Frequently with outcomes, this is a functional behavior. The object of the behavior must be something that can be *measured* or *described accurately* so that you can document when these outcomes are achieved. An example is "Pt. will demonstrate head control 100% of the time." (Behavior: demonstrate; object of the behavior: head control.)

Sometimes the behavior is implied and not specifically stated. For example, "Indep. *amb & transfers* to provide Pt. indep. mobility within his home." (Unstated behavior: demonstrate; object of the behavior: ambulation & transfers.)

Behaviors are always stated using *action verbs*. Verbs such as *be* or *know* do not describe observable or measurable activities and, therefore, are not acceptable. Instead, verbs such as *demonstrate, list,* and *state* are acceptable.

Condition

Condition includes the circumstances under which the behavior must be done or the conditions necessary for the behavior to occur. An example is "Indep. *walker* amb. *on level surfaces & curbs* for over 500 ft. × 4 within 3 wks. to allow Pt. indep. mobility @ home." A walker, level surfaces, and curbs must be available for the patient to perform this type of ambulation.

Degree

Degree is usually the portion of the outcomes that is the longest. It includes the minimal number (Example: 40 ft.), the percentage or proportion (Example: 3 out of 4 times), any limitation or departure from a fixed standard (Example: strength to 4/5 within $^1/_2$ grade), or any distinguishing features of successful performance (Example: Ⓡ LE strength equal to Ⓛ LE strength as measured by the Cybex).

When writing outcomes, the degree of performance must be *realistic, measurable,* or *observable;* must name a specific *time span* in which the outcome will be achieved; and must be *expressed in terms of function,* when possible. Discussion of the inclusion of functional terms and the setting of a time span follows.

Notice the example of an outcome given previously: "Indep walker amb on level surfaces & curbs *for over 500 feet × 4* (measurable) *within 3 wks.* (time span) *to allow Pt. indep. mobility @ home* (functional terms)."

An analysis of all of the parts of the same expected outcome follows: "Indep. walker amb. on level surfaces & curbs for over 500 ft. × 4 within 3 wks. to allow Pt. indep. mobility @ home."

A. Pt.
B. will amb. (demonstrate ambulation)
C. walker (must be present)
   on level surfaces & curbs (these surfaces must be available)
D. for over 500 ft. × 4 (measurable)
   Indep. (observable)
   within 3 wks. (time span)
   to allow Pt. indep. mobility @ home (functional)

Another example is "Pt. will be able to reach shelves in overhead cabinets @ least 6 ft. 6 in. above the floor indep. & s̄ pain within 3 wks. to allow Pt. to be able to do kitchen tasks @ home."

A. Pt.
B. will be able to reach into overhead cabinets
C. it is assumed that overhead cabinets are present
D. indep. (observable)
   @ least 6 ft. 6 in. above the floor (measurable)
   s̄ pain (measurable if you ask Pt. to rate pain on a pain scale)
   within 3 wks. (time span)
   to allow Pt. to be able to do kitchen tasks @ home (functional)

Functional Terms

Some facilities do not add the final phrase to the outcome to put it in functional terms. The advantage of using the final phrase in the previous examples is to notify third-party payers of the functional reasons for the goal. Although it may seem apparent that ambulation and reaching into overhead cabinets are useful tasks for home, this is not always so clear to others.

It is generally quite important that the expected outcomes of therapy are stated in functional terms because the ultimate goal of therapy is to make the patient more functional.

Time Span

Expected outcomes are the functional goals for the patient that have a time span of a week, a month, a year, or longer, depending on the patient's diagnosis and general condition and the therapeutic setting. The time span set is the total length of time during which the therapist will see the patient. For example, in an acute-care setting, a patient may be seen for only 3 to 5 days, whereas in certain long-term pediatric settings, a patient may be seen for a year or longer.

Setting the time span. Setting a specific time span for your expected outcomes is difficult, especially for the new practitioner, because it takes clinical experience to know how quickly a patient will progress. Even experienced therapists cannot always accurately predict the amount of time needed to achieve an outcome. Remember, expected outcomes can be revised if your patient cannot reach the outcomes within the time span set. *The Guide to Physical Therapist Practice* gives some general guidelines for number of visits, but patients may have secondary therapy diagnoses or medical diagnoses that cause the patient to fall outside of the guidelines for expected number of visits. These need to be discussed in the diagnosis part of the note. Team meetings, clinical instructors, mentors, other staff members, and class notes can serve as references for setting expected outcomes while gaining experience. Be patient with yourself as you learn to set realistic time frames.

▮ Revision

Occasionally, expected outcomes may require revision if (1) the patient's condition changes and does not allow progression to the functional level originally set, (2) the patient's condition changes and allows progression beyond the functional level originally set, or (3) the time span set is no longer appropriate and should be revised.

▮ Relationship to the Examination, Diagnosis, and Prognosis

Once the examination of a patient is complete, the therapist documents the patient's functional deficits and impairments, places them in a diagnostic category and/or practice pattern and discusses the patient's overall prognosis. Then the therapist writes expected outcomes based on the functional deficits listed, the diagnosis and the prognosis written.

To use a previous example, the following are excerpts from an initial note that you wrote (first written in Patient/Client Management Note format and then an excerpt of the SOAP Note format):

Patient/Client Management Format

HISTORY: <u>Demographics:</u> Pt. is a 65 y.o. ♂ c̄ a dx of DJD Ⓡ hip c̄ a THA on [date]... <u>Current Condition:</u> c/o Ⓡ hip pain in area of sutures of the following intensities: 7 when moving, 3 when sitting, 2 when lying still (0 = no pain, 10 = worst possible pain). Does not recall precautions for Pt.'s c̄ THA. PTA pain was constant & intensity was 9 or 10. Pt. wants to eventually return to gardening & hard work activities (Pt. goal). <u>Social Hx:</u> Lives c̄ his wife in his own home. Plans to return home c̄ his wife p̄ D/C. <u>Employment/Work:</u> Pt. is retired. <u>Living Environment:</u> Has 1 step to enter home c̄ railing on Ⓡ ascending. Owns a 3-in-1 commode, a walker, & a cane. <u>General Health Status:</u> Pt. rates general health as good; no major life changes in past yr.

Social/Health Habits: ... PTA attempted amb. for exercise daily; was only able to amb. 1 block PTA. Two yrs. ago Pt. was able to amb. 1 mi. or more. Family Hx: ... Medical/Surgical Hx: Hx of htn. Hx of hospitalization for (L) THA on 01/10/2000. Functional Status/Activity Level: Immediately PTA, PT. amb. s̄ assist. device. Hobby gardening. Gardens outside of the church. Does volunteer ushering @ church. Medications: Takes [antihypertensive medication].

SYSTEMS REVIEW: ... TESTS & MEASURES: Amb: Stood B/S c̄ walker 10% PWB (R) LE c̄ mod. assist. of 1. Transfers: Supine ↔ sit c̄ min. assist of 1. Sit ↔ stand & w/c ↔ mat pivot c̄ mod. assist. of 1. Toilet transfers not tested this date. (R) LE: Strength grossly 1/5 in hip & knee musculature; ankle dorsiflexion 4+/5; ankle plantar flexion @ least 2/5 but not tested further due to 10% PWB status. PROM: 0–20° hip flexion, 0–10° hip abduction, 0° hip extension; adduction, medial, & lateral rotation of hip not tested due to hip precautions & recent surgery. Knee flexion: 0–70°. AROM: (R) ankle WNL. Incision (R) hip 10 cm long over greater trochanter; staples intact; healing well. UEs & (L) LE: AROM WNL & strength 4+/5 throughout. Group muscle testing performed UEs; individual muscle testing performed LEs.

DIAGNOSIS: Indep. c̄ a walker is necessary for Pt. to return to home. Impairments of ↓ ROM & strength (R) LE are preventing Pt. from indep. amb. on this date. Practice Pattern: Musculoskeletal H: Impaired Joint Mobility, Motor Function, Muscle Performance & ROM Associated c̄ Joint Arthroplasty.

PROGNOSIS: Pt. has good rehab. potential. His level of function was good PTA & he has a great desire to return to a healthy, active lifestyle in the community. Should be able to return to home c̄ his wife indep. in amb. & a home exercise program to cont. to ↑ (R) LE strength & ROM p̄ 3–4 days of therapy BID.

SOAP Format

Problem: Pt. is a 65 y.o. ♂ c̄ a dx of DJD (R) hip c̄ a THA on [date]. Physician is Dr. Sienn. Hx of htn. Hx of hospitalization for (L) THA on 01/10/2000. Takes [antihypertensive medication]. Pt. is (R)-hand dominant.

S: CURRENT CONDITION: c/o (R) hip pain in area of sutures of the following intensities: 7 when moving, 3 when sitting, 2 when lying still (0 = no pain, 10 = worst possible pain). Does not recall precautions for Pt.'s c̄ THA. PTA pain was constant & intensity was 9 or 10. PT. GOALS: Pt. wants to eventually return to gardening & hard work activities (Pt. goal). SOCIAL HX: Lives c̄ his wife in his own home. Plans to return home c̄ his wife p̄ D/C. EMPLOYMENT/WORK: Pt. is retired. LIVING ENVIRONMENT: Has 1 step to enter home c̄ railing on (R) ascending. Owns a 3-in-1 commode, a walker, & a cane. GENERAL HEALTH STATUS: Pt. rates general health as good; no major life changes in past yr. SOCIAL/HEALTH HABITS: ... PTA attempted amb. for exercise daily; was only able to amb. 1 block PTA. Two yrs. ago Pt. was able to amb. 1 mi. or more. FAMILY HX: ... FUNCTIONAL STATUS/ACTIVITY LEVEL: Immediately PTA, PT. amb. s̄ assist. device. Hobby gardening. Gardens outside of the church. Does volunteer ushering @ church.

O: SYSTEMS REVIEW: ... TRANSFERS: Supine ↔ sit c̄ min. assist. of 1. Sit ↔ stand & w/c ↔ mat pivot c̄ mod. assist. of 1. Toilet transfers not tested this date. (R) LE: Strength grossly 1/5 in hip & knee musculature; ankle dorsiflexion 4+/5; ankle plantar flexion @ least 2/5 but not tested further due to 10% PWB status. PROM: 0–20° hip flexion, 0–10° hip abduction, 0° hip extension; adduction, medical & lateral rotation of hip not tested due to hip precautions & recent surgery. Knee flexion: 0–70°. AROM: (R) ankle WNL. Incision (R) hip 10 cm long over greater trochanter; staples intact; healing well. UE & (L) LE: AROM WNL & strength 4+/5 throughout bilat. UEs & (L) LE. Group muscle testing performed UEs; individual muscle testing performed LEs.

A: DIAGNOSIS: Indep. c̄ a walker is necessary for Pt. to return to home. Impairments of ↓ ROM & strength (R) LE are preventing Pt. from indep. amb. on this date. Practice Pattern: Musculoskeletal H: Impaired Joint Mobility, Motor Function, Muscle Performance & ROM Associated c̄ Joint Arthroplasty. PROGNOSIS: Pt. has good rehab. potential. His level of function was good PTA & he has a great desire to return to a healthy, active lifestyle in the community. Should be able to return to home c̄ his wife indep. in amb. & home exercise program to cont. to ↑ (R) LE strength & ROM p̄ 3–4 days of therapy BID.

The expected outcomes (what will be achieved by the time the patient is discharged from the hospital in 3 days) are as follows:

1. Indep. transfers on/off toilet, supine ↔ sit, sit ↔ stand, chair ↔ bed, so Pt. is safe for ADL @ home within 3 days. (This covers the functional deficit concerning transfers.)
2. Indep. walker amb. FWB (R) LE for @ least 150 ft. × 2 on level surfaces & on 1 step so Pt. can func-

tion indep in amb. @ home within 3 days. (This covers the functional deficit concerning ambulation.)

Setting Priorities

Expected outcomes are listed in order of priority. Often, the most important or more vital functional activity is listed first. In the previous example, transfers were listed first because a patient can perform safe transfers and must do so whether or not the patient is independent in ambulation. For the purposes of this workbook, you are not expected to set expected outcome priorities. You will be guided on what the outcomes should be and how to set priorities.

Relationship to Anticipated Goals

Anticipated goals are written as steps along the way to achieving expected outcomes.

E X A M P L E

Expected Outcome

Indep. amb. c̄ a walker FWB Ⓡ LE for @ least 150 ft. × 2 on level surfaces & on 1 step elevation within 1 mo. to allow Pt. to amb. around her house.

Anticipated Goal

Pt. will amb. 30 ft. × 2 in // bars 10% PWB Ⓡ LE within 3 days c̄ mod. + 1 assist.

Anticipated Goal (Later in the Patient's Progress)

Pt. will amb. c̄ a walker 50 ft. × 2 10% PWB Ⓡ LE within 1 wk. c̄ min. + 1 assist.

Anticipated goals also address impairments that affect the patient's ability to perform functional activities, such as range of motion and strength affecting ambulation and transfers for patients who have had a total joint arthroplasty.

As you can see in the following example, the anticipated goals include educational goals and goals that address the impairments. Notice that the first anticipated goal in the example specifically tied the impairment with the functional activity involved. To summarize, anticipated goals can

---

E X A M P L E

(Using the previous case)

Expected Outcome

1. Indep. transfers on/off toilet, supine ↔ sit, sit ↔ stand, chair ↔ bed, so Pt. is safe for ADL @ home within 3 days. (This covers the functional deficit concerning transfers.)

Anticipated Goals

1. Pt. will ↑ Ⓡ hip flexion AROM to 0–80° within 3 days to assist. c̄ indep. transfers.
2. Pt. will perform home exercise program to ↑ Ⓡ hip & knee AROM & strength indep. within 3 days.
3. Pt. will ↑ strength Ⓡ hip abduction and flexion to @ least 3/5 within 3 days to assist. c̄ indep. transfers and amb.

---

address issues of function, impairments and education for the patient that are implied or stated in the expected outcomes.

A Word About Interim Notes

When writing an interim note, expected outcomes are usually not addressed unless they are achieved or need to be revised.

A Word About Discharge Summaries

When writing a discharge summary, list the expected outcomes and most recent anticipated goals, indicating which expected outcomes and anticipated goals have been achieved and which have not been achieved. This is particularly important for expected outcomes because expected outcomes by definition list the functional status the patient is to achieve by discharge.

Summary

Outcomes state the long-term plans for the patient. It is important that they are structured and clearly defined. They are based on the examination, therapy diagnosis, and prognosis. Expected outcomes require the clinical judgment of the therapist to set the parameters of each goal. Often expected outcomes are functional in nature, whereas anticipated goals address both function and impairments.

The worksheets that follow will assist you in setting expected outcomes and give you practice in writing outcomes. They will also let you analyze several outcomes, letting you see how each outcome is structured correctly. After you review the previous material, complete the worksheets, and compare your work to the answers in Appendix A, you should be able to write an expected outcome correctly when given the parameters, recognize when an expected outcome is incomplete, and state the components missing from an incomplete expected outcome.

▌Acknowledgment

Instructional Objectives, by the Teaching Improvement Project Systems for Health Care Educators (Center for Learning Resources, College of Allied Health Professions, University of Kentucky, Lexington, KY, 40536-0218) was very helpful in the preparation of this chapter.

Writing Expected Outcomes (Long-Term Goals):

Worksheet 1

 PART I. In each of the following examples, identify the (A) audience, (B) behavior, (C) condition, and (D) degree.

1. Indep. w/c management & propulsion for approx. 50 ft. × 10 at home within 1 mo.

    A. _____

    B. _____

    C. _____

    D. _____

    _____

    _____

    _____

2. Within 2 wks. Pt. will demonstrate indep. amb. c̄ prosthesis s̄ device on at least 14 stairs & for at least $^1/_2$ mi. on even & uneven surfaces to assure Pt.'s ability to amb. in & out of his home & around his yard.

    A. _____

    B. _____

    C. _____

    D. _____

    _____

    _____

    _____

    _____

3. Pt. will demonstrate good body mechanics while lifting up to 50 lbs. in order to allow Pt. to return to work fully functional @ performing his job within 4 wks. of Rx.

    A. _____

    B. _____

    C. _____

    D. _____

    _____

    _____

    _____

4. Pt. will demonstrate indep. segmental rolling $\bar{p}$ 6 mo. of Rx in order to make Pt. more functional as she sleeps & plays.

A. _____

B. _____

C. _____

D. _____

_____

_____

PART II. Given the following components of an expected outcome, write them into an expected outcome.

1. A. Pt.

    B. will amb. (will demonstrate amb.)

    C. $\bar{c}$ crutches,

        on level surfaces & 1 step elevation,

        NWB Ⓛ LE

    D. indep. (observable)

        $\bar{p}$ 2 days (time span)

        40 ft. $\times$ 3 (measurable)

        to allow Pt. to get around her house for ADL (functional)

    Expected Outcome: _____

    _____

    _____

    _____

    _____

    _____

    _____

    _____

    _____

    _____

2. A. Pt.

    B. will demonstrate care & wrapping of her residual limb

    C. $\bar{c}$ elastic wrap

    D. indep. (observable)

        applying even pressure (observable)

        100% of the time (measurable)

        to prepare for prosthetic training

        (functional)

        within 3 days (time span)

    Expected Outcome: _____

    _____

    _____

    _____

    _____

    _____

    _____

    _____

3. A. Pt.   Expected Outcome: _____

   B. will be able to lift a box   _____

   C. from an overhead cupboard &   _____

       place it on a table   _____

   D. using bilat. UEs equally   _____
       (observable)   _____

       within 2 mo. (time span)   _____

       in order to enable Pt.'s ability to   _____
       reach items on the shelves in her
       kitchen & closets @ home during   _____
       ADL (functional)   _____

       box will be 5 lbs. (measurable)   _____

4. A. Pt.   Expected Outcome: _____

   B. will amb.   _____

   C. in her home   _____

   D. $\bar{s}$ device   _____

       for 50 ft. × 4 (measurable)   _____

       using pursed lip breathing pattern   _____

         (observable)   _____

       to enable her to cook & perform   _____
       ADLs (functional)   _____

       within 4 wks. of Rx.   _____

PART III. Write the appropriate expected outcomes as described below.

DIAGNOSIS: Pt.'s inability to lift pots & pans in her kitchen & inability to reach items in her overhead kitchen cabinets is caused by ↓ Ⓡ elbow flexion and extension AROM & ↓ Ⓡ biceps and triceps strength. Practice Pattern: Musculoskeletal G—Impaired Joint Mobility, Muscle Performance, and ROM Associated $\bar{c}$ Fx. PROGNOSIS: Pt. has good rehab. potential. Should improve quickly, within 10 visits, with follow up of Pt. performing home exercise program between visits.

Use the instructions below to formulate an expected outcome for each functional deficit mentioned.

1. The Pt. is unable to lift pots & pans in her kitchen. You judge that by D/C, the Pt. should be able to lift pots & pans up to 20 pounds.

   Expected Outcome: _____

   _____

   _____

   _____

2. The Pt. is unable to reach items in her overhead kitchen cabinets. You judge that by D/C the Pt. should be able to reach items in overhead cabinets up to 5 ft. 10 in.

Expected Outcome: _____

_____

_____

_____

Answers to "Writing Expected Outcomes: Worksheet 1" are provided in Appendix A.

Writing Expected Outcomes (Long-Term Goals):
Worksheet 2

PART I. In each of the following examples, identify the (A) audience, (B) behavior, (C) condition, and (D) degree.

1. Indep. amb. c̄ straight cane for 150 ft. × 2 on level surfaces & on @ least 5 stairs within 1 wk. so Pt.'s level of indep. @ home ↑.

   A. _____

   B. _____

   C. _____

   D. _____

   _____

   _____

2. Pt.'s wife will indep. transfer Pt. w/c ↔ supine in bed & w/c ↔ toilet giving min. + 1 assist. to Pt. p̄ 1 mo. of Rx & 5 sessions of family teaching so wife can care for Pt. @ home.

   A. _____

   B. _____

   C. _____

   D. _____

   _____

   _____

   _____

3. Indep. transfers w/c ↔ floor within 3 mo. of Rx so Pt. can safely play on the floor c̄ her siblings.

   A. _____

   B. _____

   C. _____

   D. _____

   _____

   _____

PART II. Given the following components of an expected outcome, write them into the expected outcome.

1. A. Pt.
    B. will sit
    C. on the edge of a mat or chair
    D. s̄ falling (observable)
        for @ least 10 min. (measurable)
        p̄ 2 mo. of Rx (time span)
        to allow Pt. to more safely function
            @ school (function)

    Expected Outcome: _____
    _____
    _____
    _____
    _____
    _____
    _____

2. A. Pt.
    B. will demonstrate transfers
        supine ↔ sit, sit ↔ stand,
        on/off toilet
    C. toilet c̄ raised toilet seat &
        some surface (mat or bed)
        on which to lie are necessary
    D. independent (observable)
        p̄ 2 wks. of Rx (time span)
        in order for Pt. to function indep.
            @ home (function)

    Expected Outcome: _____
    _____
    _____
    _____
    _____
    _____
    _____
    _____
    _____

3. A. Pt.
    B. will demonstrate w/c propulsion
    C. on level surfaces including tiled
        and carpeted surfaces
    D. independently (observable)
        after one month of therapy
            (time span)
        to increase Pt.'s independence
            at home (functional)

    Expected Outcome: _____
    _____
    _____
    _____
    _____
    _____
    _____
    _____

PART III. Write the expected outcomes as described below.

Case

You have just completed writing the examination portions of a note.

DIAGNOSIS: Pt.'s gait deviations are caused by ↓ ROM Ⓛ knee & ↓ strength Ⓛ quadriceps. Pt. is not indep. & safe in amb. c̄ walker & transfers so Pt. cannot return to home @ this time because he lives alone. <u>Practice Pattern:</u> Musculoskeletal H—Impaired Joint Mobility, Motor Function, Muscle Performance, & ROM Associated c̄ Joint Arthroplasty. PROGNOSIS: Pt. has good rehab. potential & should be able to return to home. Residual deficits in Ⓡ LE from stroke 2 yrs. ago may lengthen rehab. time. Anticipate 2 wk. stay on SNF Unit to prepare Pt. to be fully functional & safe at home.

Use the following instructions to formulate an expected outcome for each functional deficit mentioned.

EXPECTED OUTCOMES:

1. The patient is not safe in ambulation. You believe patient will ambulate with a walker on level surfaces and 3 stairs with a handrail full weight bearing as tolerated in by discharge in 2 weeks.

   <u>Expected Outcome:</u> _____

   _____

   _____

   _____

2. The patient is unable to transfer independently. You judge that by discharge the patient should be able to transfer bed to/from chair, sit to/from stand, on/off commode independently.

   <u>Expected Outcome:</u> _____

   _____

   _____

   _____

Answers to "Writing Expected Outcomes: Worksheet 2" are provided in Appendix A.

CHAPTER 14

Writing Anticipated Goals (Short-Term Goals)

Anticipated goals are part of the Plan of Care portion of the note. They are the interim steps along the way to achieving expected outcomes (which are the final product of therapeutic intervention). Once the expected outcomes of therapy have been determined, the anticipated goals are then set. The specific regimen of interventions is designed to achieve the anticipated goals.

▮ Reasons for Writing Goals

Anticipated goals are written (1) to direct interventions to the specific needs and problems of the patients, (2) to set priorities in interventions and measure the effectiveness of interventions, (3) to assist with cost effectiveness (for purposes of third-party payment), and (4) to communicate therapy goals to other health-care professionals. Anticipated goals help to guide the immediate intervention plan. Periodically reviewing and resetting anticipated goals helps the therapist and the patient realize the progress that the patient has made.

▮ The Structure of Anticipated Goals

Like Expected Outcomes, Anticipated Goals are objectives, and need to contain the following elements that a good objective contains:

A. Audience

B. Behavior

C. Condition

D. Degree

A brief review of the definitions of the elements of a goal with examples from anticipated goals follows.

Audience

Almost always, the audience is the patient. However, it *can* be a family member, as in "Pt.'s wife will wrap Pt.'s residual limb c̄ 3-in. elastic wrap c̄ verbal cues only p̄ 4 visits to prepare Pt. for prosthetic training." Often the audience is implied in goal writing, and it is not necessary to say, "Pt. will demonstrate ..." or "Pt. will be ..."

Behavior

This is always indicated by a verb followed by the object of the behavior. Good examples are "↑ ℝ knee AROM ...," "↓ dependence in dressing," and "improve gait pattern ..." The object of the behavior must be something that can be *measured* or *described accurately* so that an increase or improvement can be documented at a later date.

Condition

Condition includes the circumstances under which the behavior must be done. Examples are "↓ dependence in *walker* amb. to min + 1 assist. within 1 wk.," "indep. amb. s̄ *assistive device on level surfaces* for 10 ft. × 2 within 1 wk."

Sometimes the circumstances under which the behavior must be done are implied. If "Normal pain-free ℝ LE AROM & strength" is set as an outcome, it is implied that you must have a goniometer available and strength will be measured via manual muscle testing.

Degree

Degree includes the minimal number, the percentage or proportion, any limitation or departure from a fixed standard, or any distinguishing features of successful performance.

When writing goals, the degree of performance must be *realistic, measurable,* or *observable;* must name a specific *time span;* and should *tie into functional activities* whenever possible.

Consider the example of a goal given previously: "Pt.'s wife will wrap Pt.'s residual limb $\bar{c}$ 3-in. elastic wrap $\bar{c}$ *verbal cues only* (measurable) $\bar{p}$ *4 visits* (time span) *to prepare Pt. for prosthetic training* (functional terms)."

Review this goal and analyze its parts: "Pt.'s wife will wrap Pt.'s residual limb $\bar{c}$ 3-in. elastic wrap $\bar{c}$ verbal cues only $\bar{p}$ 4 visits to prepare Pt. for prosthetic training."

A. Pt.'s wife
B. will wrap Pt.'s residual limb
C. 3-in. elastic wrap
D. $\bar{c}$ verbal cues only (observable)
    $\bar{p}$ 4 visits (time span)
    to prepare Pt. for prosthetic training (functional)

Another example follows: "↑ AROM ⑀ knee flexion to 5–55° within 3 days to improve transfers & gait."

A. Pt. (implied)
B. will ↑ ⑀ knee flexion AROM
C. no conditions given (assumed: goniometer will be used)
D. 5–55° (measurable)
    within 3 days (time span)
    to improve Pt.'s transfers & gait (functional)

Functional Terms

Therapists at some facilities do not add the final phrase to the goal to put it in functional terms. The advantage of using the final phrase in the previous examples is to notify third-party payers of the functional reasons for the goal. Among professionals, it is generally known that he patient will not be very functional in transfers and ambulation with a knee with very little AROM; however, this is not always so clear to others. The goal of wrapping the residual limb is not always clear to all personnel working with the patient and certainly could confuse third-party payers if this is one of the patient's goals. Including functional terms is becoming increasingly normative when writing all goals.

If an explanation of a goal is needed and stating the goal in functional terms is not adequate to explain the reasons for setting the goal, it should be explained further under the Prognosis or Diagnosis part of the note.

Although anticipated goals are not written in functional terms at all facilities, the importance of using functional terms is rapidly increasing. Some therapists assume that if the expected outcomes are functional and the anticipated goals correspond well with the expected outcomes, then the functional reasons for the anticipated goals are obvious. However, the relationship between the expected outcomes and anticipated goals is not as obvious as therapists may assume. Other therapists always use function and only state anticipated goals in functional terms. This varies from facility to facility. You will adapt your style of writing anticipated goals as you adapt to various clinical settings.

Clarity

Poorly written anticipated goals do not clearly communicate the purpose of therapy for the patient. If certain components of a well-written goal are not included (such as time span, functional terms, or measurable terms), the purpose of interventions may be very unclear. The lack of clarity will be especially confusing to third-party payers and health care professionals who are not familiar with therapy interventions and their purposes. At times, the goal must be related to patient function for the purpose of communicating clearly to those reading the patient care note.

Time Span

Anticipated goals are patient objectives that have a time span for their achievement. This can be a few days or a week or longer, depending on the patient's diagnosis and general condition. For example, a patient with a brain injury may take 3 to 4 months for rehabilitation at times, so anticipated goals can be set weekly or occasionally for a 2-week period. Other patients in some pediatric settings may have expected outcomes set for 1 year and anticipated goals may be set for 1 to 3 months.

Setting the time span. Setting a specific time span in which a goal will be achieved is difficult, especially for new practitioners, because it takes clinical experience to know how quickly a patient will progress. At times, even experienced clinicians have difficulty predicting how quickly a patient should progress. Generally, a clinician can consider when a note on a particular patient must be written again and what the patient's status will be at that time. If the patient's status will change by the time a note is due to be written, the time span can be set to correspond with the date the note is due. If achieving a goal will take longer, choose a longer time span. If it will take less time, set a shorter time span.

Remember, anticipated goals can always be revised if the time span set is not correct. Clinical instructors, peers, *The Guide to Physical Therapist Practice,** and class notes can serve as references for setting realistic time spans.

At times, anticipated goals are not necessary because of an anticipated extremely short patient length of stay. For example, if the patient is only to be seen by a therapist one or two times, the expected outcomes may be adequate and anticipated goals are not needed. If the expected outcomes imply or require an improvement at the impairment level, anticipated goals may be set if the expected outcomes written are purely functional.

▌Revision

Anticipated goals must be revised periodically. An anticipated goal should be revised if (1) the period mentioned in the goal has passed, or (2) the patient has achieved the goals set. Consider a previous example:

↓ dependence in walker amb. to min. +1 assist. for 10 ft. × 2 within 1 wk. to facilitate indep. walker amb. at home.

Assume 3 days have passed and the patient required minimal of 1 assistance and is progressing. The goal is reset to read:

↓ dependence in walker amb. to SBA for 60 ft. × 4 within 1 wk. to facilitate amb. functional distances needed for home.

Another week passes and the patient's rate of progress has decreased. The therapist now comments on lack of progress and resets the anticipated goal:

Goal to ↓ amb. dependence not yet achieved due to … (it is good to give a reason if there is one.) Will ↓ dependence in amb. c̄ walker to SBA for 60 ft. × 4 within 1 more wk. of Rx.

▌Relationship to Expected Outcomes

Anticipated goals are written as steps along the way to achieving expected outcomes. Please see the first example.

Anticipated goals also address impairments that affect the patient's ability to perform functional activities, such as range of motion and strength affecting ambulation and transfers for patients who have had a total joint arthroplasty.

As you can see in the second example, the anticipated goals include educational goals and goals that

The Guide to Physical Therapist Practice.

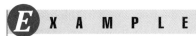

E X A M P L E

Expected Outcome

Indep. amb. c̄ a walker FWB Ⓡ LE for @ least 150 ft. × 2 on level surfaces & on 1 step elevation within 1 mo. to allow Pt. to amb. around her house.

Anticipated Goal

Pt. will amb. 30 ft. × 2 in // bars 10% PWB Ⓡ LE within 3 days c̄ mod. + 1 assist.

Anticipated Goal (Later on in the Patient's Progress)

Pt. will amb. c̄ a walker 50 ft. × 2 10% PWB Ⓡ LE within 1 wk. c̄ min. + 1 assist.

E X A M P L E

Using the previous case

Expected Outcome

1. Indep. transfers on/off toilet, supine ↔ sit, sit ↔ stand, chair ↔ bed, so Pt. is safe for ADL @ home within 3 days. (This covers the functional deficit concerning transfers.)

Anticipated Goals

1. Pt. will ↑ Ⓡ hip flexion AROM to 0–80° within 3 days to assist. c̄ indep. transfers.
2. Pt. will perform home exercise program to ↑Ⓡ hip & knee AROM & strength indep. within 3 days.
3. Pt. will ↑ strength Ⓡ hip abduction and flexion to @ least 3/5 within 3 days to assist. c̄ indep. transfers and amb.

address the impairments. Notice that the first anticipated goal in the example specifically tied the impairment with the functional activity involved. In summary, anticipated goals can address issues of function, impairments, and education for the patient that are implied or stated in the expected outcomes.

▌Setting Priorities

Priorities are set for anticipated goals by looking at the priorities set for the expected outcomes. If the expected outcomes are listed in order of priority and the anticipated goals are set to meet the expected outcomes, the anticipated goals already have a priority order. If there is more than one anticipated goal for a particular expected outcome, as in the previous example, the anticipated goals for that outcome are listed with the most functional goal (such as ambulation or transfers) listed first. Anticipated goals that address impairments (such as range of motion or strength) usually follow more functional anticipated goals.

For the purposes of this workbook, you are not expected to set goal priorities. You will be guided in setting the goals and in setting goal priorities if the priorities are different from those of the expected outcomes or if there are two or more anticipated goals that correspond to one expected outcome.

Relationship to the Intervention Plan

When anticipated goals are set, the therapist (with the patient's input) determines the interventions for the next few days. When an intervention plan is set up, an intervention to work toward *each* of the anticipated goals must be included.

E X A M P L E

Expected Outcomes
1. Indep. walker amb. on level surfaces FWB for 70 ft. × 2 & on 1 step within 2 wks. so Pt. can get in & out of her home & amb. within her home safely.
2. Indep. transfers chair ↔ bed, sit ↔ stand, on/off toilet within 2 wks. so Pt. can function indep. & safely @ home.

Anticipated Goals
1. Pt. will amb. c̄ walker 50% PWB Ⓡ LE for ~20 ft. × 2 within 1 wk. to facilitate amb. @ home (*from first expected outcome*).
2. Pt. will transfer bed ↔ chair & sit ↔ stand c̄ min. assist of 1 in 1 wk. (*from second expected outcome*).
3. Pt. will ↑ Ⓡ quadriceps strength to @ least 2/5 within 1 wk. to ↑ indep. in amb. & transfers (*from first and second expected outcomes*).
4. Pt. will indep. demonstrate exercises that he is to perform in the hospital room within 2 Rx sessions to ↑ amb. indep. (*from first and second expected outcomes*).

Intervention Plan
BID @ B/S: Amb. training c̄ a walker, beginning c̄ 50% PWB & progressing to wt. bearing & distance as tolerated (from first anticipated goal). Transfer training, beginning c̄ bed ↔ chair & sit ↔ stand & progressing to on/off toilet (*from second anticipated goal—placed second in priority because it is*

functional). Pt. will be given written & verbal instruction in exercise program to be performed in the hospital room between Rx sessions (attached) (from fourth anticipated goal). AAROM progressing to AROM exercises Ⓡ knee, emphasizing quadriceps functioning (*from third anticipated goal*).

Sometimes an intervention works toward more than one anticipated goal at a time, as demonstrated in the previous example. Further explanation of the relationship of the intervention plan to the anticipated goals is discussed in Chapter 15.

Anticipated Goals in Interim (Progress) Notes

When writing an interim note, the therapist refers to the anticipated goals previously set and sets new anticipated goals if the previous anticipated goals have been achieved. If an anticipated goal previously set has not yet been achieved, the therapist comments on the reason it has not yet been achieved. Then the therapist either resets the goal to make it more reasonable or restates the goal as a goal to be achieved by the next interim note to be written.

E X A M P L E

1. ANTICIPATED GOALS: Goal #4 of (date) not yet achieved due to ↓ in Pt.'s medical status; will cont. to work toward same goal for 1 more wk.
2. ANTICIPATED GOALS: All achieved. Will work directly toward expected outcomes set on (date).

Anticipated Goals in Discharge Notes

When writing a discharge summary, the therapist may comment on the most recently set anticipated goals as to whether or not they were achieved and why. However, in a discharge summary, the emphasis should be on the expected outcomes and why they were or were not achieved.

Summary

Setting anticipated goals is the second step in the Plan of Care part of the note. It is the fifth step in the overall examination, evaluation, and planning process for the patient. Anticipated goals are based on the expected outcomes and direct the immediate course of the intervention plan. The period covered by anticipated goals is briefer than that for expected outcomes. Revision of anticipated goals is done on a regular basis and generally indicates that the patient is making progress. Setting anticipated goals involves professional judgment.

The worksheets that follow will assist you in setting anticipated goals and give you practice in writing the goals. They will also let you analyze several goals, allowing you to see how each goal is structured. After reviewing the previous material, completing the worksheets, and comparing your work to the answers in Appendix A, you should be able to write an anticipated goal correctly when given the parameters of the goal, recognize when a goal is incomplete, and state the components missing from an incomplete anticipated goal.

▌Acknowledgment

Instructional Objectives, by the Teaching Improvement Project Systems for Health Care Educators (Center for Learning Resources, College of Allied Health Professions, University of Kentucky, Lexington, KY, 40536-0218) was very helpful in the preparation of this chapter.

Writing Anticipated Goals (Short-Term Goals):

Worksheet 1

PART I. In each of the following examples, identify the audience (A), behavior (B), condition (C), and degree (D).

1. ANTICIPATED GOAL: ↑ Ⓡ shoulder flexion AROM to 0–90° within 6 Rx sessions to work toward Pt. reaching her overhead kitchen cupboards.

   A. _____

   B. _____

   C. _____

   D. _____

   _____

   _____

   _____

2. ANTICIPATED GOAL: Pt. will grasp object in midline 3 out of 4 times within 3 mo. in order to ↑ Pt's functional use of his UEs during ADLs.

   A. _____

   B. _____

   C. _____

   D. _____

   _____

   _____

   _____

3. ANTICIPATED GOAL: Pt. will demonstrate good body mechanics by correct performance of at least 90% of tasks in obstacle course p̄ 3 Rx sessions to prevent further Pt. injury @ work.

   A. _____

   B. _____

   C. _____

   D. _____

   _____

   _____

   _____

PART II. Given the following components of a goal, write them into an anticipated goal.

1. A. Pt.

    B. will ↓ dependence in amb.

    C. using a walker

        on level surfaces only

        NWB Ⓛ LE

    D. ~100 ft. × 2

        1 wk. of Rx

        independent

Anticipated Goal: _____

_____

_____

_____

_____

_____

_____

2. A. Pt.'s wife & son

    B. transfer Pt. w/c ↔ supine in bed

    C. bed & w/c are necessary

    D. independently

        p̄ 4 family training sessions

        to care for Pt. @ home

Anticipated Goal: _____

_____

_____

_____

_____

_____

3. A. Pt.

    B. wrap residual limb

    C. 3 in. elastic wrap

    D. c̄ verbal cues for placement of

        elastic wrap

        after 5 Rx sessions

        to prepare for prosthetic training

Anticipated Goal: _____

_____

_____

_____

_____

_____

_____

 PART III. In each of the following cases, write the appropriate anticipated goal.

1. **Case 1**

    TESTS & MEASURES (O): Requires verbal cues & mod + 1 assist.
    DIAGNOSIS & PROGNOSIS: ...
    EXPECTED OUTCOME: Indep. donning/doffing prosthesis in 1 wk. to allow Pt. to come to standing.
    ANTICIPATED GOAL: _____

    _____

    You judge that 1 week from now only standby assistance of one person and no verbal cues will be needed.

2. **Case 2**

MEDICAL DX: stroke c̄ (L) sided weakness.
TESTS & MEASURES (O): <u>Amb</u>: Stands in // bars c̄ mod + 1 assist. & verbal cues for wt. shift. Wt. shift onto (L) LE is poor; Pt. bears only 10 lbs. of wt. on (L) LE.
DIAGNOSIS & PROGNOSIS: ...
EXPECTED OUTCOME: Indep. amb. c̄ straight cane for unlimited distances c̄ normal gait pattern, including normal wt. shift onto (L) LE.
ANTICIPATED GOAL: _____

_____

You judge that in 1 week minimal assistance of one person and verbal cues will be needed for the patient to be able to stand in the parallel bars with at least half of his body weight shifted onto his left leg.

3. **Case 3**

MEDICAL DX: L4 herniated disc. Lumbar laminectomy performed on (date).
TESTS & MEASURES (O): <u>Trunk:</u> Can tolerate lying prone for 5 min. Cannot tolerate further trunk extension.
EXPECTEDOUTCOME Pt. will be able to perform all ADLs s̄ pain p̄ 8 Rx.
ANTICIPATED GOAL: _____

_____

You judge that after 2 Rx sessions the patient will be pain free in the prone-on elbow position for 5 min.

PART IV. State which components each of the following anticipated goals are missing.

1. ANTICIPATED GOAL: Pt. will be able to perform sliding board transfers.

Answer: _____

_____

2. ANTICIPATED GOAL: Pt. will demonstrate the correct position for hip flexor stretching.

Answer: _____

_____

3. ANTICIPATED GOAL: 10-min. exercise routine s̄ fatigue within 5 wks.

Answer: _____

_____

Answers to "Writing Anticipated Goals: Worksheet 1" are provided in Appendix A.

Writing Anticipated Goals (Short-Term Goals):

Worksheet 2

PART I. In each of the following examples, identify the audience (A), behavior (B), condition (C), and degree (D).

1. ANTICIPATED GOAL: p̄ 6 Rx sessions, Pt. will ↑ cardiopulmonary endurance as demonstrated by max. ↑ resp. rate of 5/min. p̄ amb. s̄ device for 150 ft. to ↑ Pt. function @ home.

   A. _____

   B. _____

   C. _____

   D. _____

   _____

   _____

2. ANTICIPATED GOAL: Pt. will able to long sit propped c̄ a pillow or wedge maintaining good head position 0–45° of neck flexion for 1 min. p̄ 6 wks. of Rx to assist. c̄ Pt. function in the classroom.

   A. _____

   B. _____

   C. _____

   D. _____

   _____

   _____

3. ANTICIPATED GOAL: Pt. will transfer supine ↔ sit on a mat using rotation & pushing c̄ his UEs (1 out of 3 attempts correct) within 1 mo.

   A. _____

   B. _____

   C. _____

   D. _____

   _____

   _____

PART II. Given the following components of a goal, write them into an anticipated goal.

1. A. Pt.

   B. hold head

   C. while Pt. is supine

   D. in midline

      15 sec.

      within 3 mo. of Rx

      to assist Pt.'s ability to learn

   Anticipated Goal: _____

   _____

   _____

   _____

   _____

2. A. Pt.

   B. rolling supine ↔ prone

   C. on a mat

   D. in 6–8 wks.

      independently

      to assist c̄ indep ADLs

   Anticipated Goal: _____

   _____

   _____

   _____

   _____

3. A. Pt.

   B. ambulate stairs with walker

   C. walker & stairs must be

         available

      50% PWB Ⓡ LE

   D. 5 stairs

      c̄ min. assist. from his wife

      independently

      1 week

      to ↑ Pt. function at home

   Anticipated Goal: _____

   _____

   _____

   _____

   _____

   _____

   _____

 PART III. In each of the following excerpted cases, write the appropriate anticipated goal.

1. **Case 1**

   MEDICAL DX: COPD; respiratory failure.

   TESTS & MEASURES (O): <u>Functional use of UEs:</u> Unable to take any items out of overhead cupboards. <u>Strength:</u> 3/5 throughout UEs bilat. <u>AROM:</u> Limited to 90° of Ⓡ shoulder flex. & 80° Ⓛ shoulder flex ... Endurance: c̄ 5 reps. of bilat. UE PNF diagonals, Pt's pulse ↑ by 20 beats/min.

   DIAGNOSIS & PROGNOSIS: ...

   EXPECTED OUTCOME: Pt. will be able to retrieve items 5 lbs. in weight from upper shelf over overhead cabinet.

   ANTICIPATED GOAL: _____

   _____

_____
_____
_____
_____
_____
_____
_____
_____
_____
_____
_____
_____
_____
_____
_____

1. You judge that the patient will perform 7 repetitions of each of the 2 PNF patterns for the arms after 1 wk. of Rx within available AROM.

2. You judge that AROM of Ⓡ shoulder flexion will ↑ to 100° within 1 wk. of Rx.

3. You judge that AROM of Ⓛ shoulder flexion will ↑ to 90° within 1 wk. of Rx.

4. You judge that the strength throughout the bilat. UEs will ↑ to 3+/5 bilat. within available AROM after 1 wk. of Rx.

5. You judge that the Pt. will be able to retrieve items 0.5 lbs. in wt. from the lower shelf of overhead cabinet after 1 wk. of Rx.

2. **Case 2**

MEDICAL DX: whiplash.
HISTORY (S): <u>Current condition:</u> c/o neck pain of an intensity of 9 (0 = no pain, 10 = worst possible pain) c̄ any movement of the neck.
TESTS & MEASURES (O): <u>AROM:</u> 0–5° cervical rotation Ⓛ & Ⓡ.
DIAGNOSIS & PROGNOSIS: …
EXPECTED OUTCOME: Pt. will be pain free in cervical area & functional in all ADLs.
ANTICIPATED GOAL: _____

_____

You judge that the patient will be able to move her head to about 10° of rotation to either side in 2 days.

3. **Case 3**

MEDICAL DX: Fx Ⓡ tibial plateau. Long leg cast applied (date).
TESTS & MEASURES (O): <u>Amb.:</u> c̄ walker 40 ft. × 1 NWB Ⓡ LE c̄ mod. + 1 assist.
EXPECTED OUTCOMES: Indep. amb. c̄ crutches for 200 ft. × 4 NWB Ⓡ LE on level surfaces & stairs within 2 wks. of Rx.
ANTICIPATED GOAL: _____

_____

You judge that the patient will be able to ambulate 40 ft. twice on level surfaces in 1 wk. but will still require minimal assistance of 1 person to ambulate.

PART IV. State which components of each of the following anticipated goals are missing.

1. ANTICIPATED GOALS: ↓ dependence in amb. to min. + 1 c̄ walker 40 ft. × 2 NWB Ⓡ LE.

Answer: _____

_____

_____

2. ANTICIPATED GOALS: ↑ Ⓡ shoulder abduction AROM within 3 days.

Answer: _____

_____

3. ANTICIPATED GOALS: ↑ & ↓ stairs c̄ min. + 1 assist.

Answer: _____

_____

Answers to "Writing Anticipated Goals: Worksheet 2" are provided in Appendix A.

Documenting Planned Interventions

The *Intervention Plan* portion of the note is the final part of the Plan of Care. It contains a plan for the interventions that the patient will receive while in therapy. One or more interventions exist to achieve each of the anticipated goals. Certain information must be included in the intervention plan section of the note, just as certain information is needed for documentation of the examination to be complete.

Information Included Under the Plan

The following information *must be* included in the *Intervention Plan* section of a note:

- Frequency per day or per week that the patient will be seen

- The interventions that the patient will receive (The amount of specificity may depend on the setting. See the following text for more detail on describing intervention. For purposes of these worksheets, a significant level of detail is expected.)

- If a discharge note, where the patient is going and the number of times the patient was seen in therapy

The following are also frequently included in the plan section:

- The location of the treatment (at bedside, in the department, in a pool, at home)

- The treatment progression

- Plans for further assessment or reassessment

- Plans for discharge

- Patient and family education (e.g., home program plans or what was taught to the patient or the patient's family—attach a copy of any home pro-

grams [signed and dated, of course] to the note, if possible)

- Equipment needs and equipment ordered for or sold to the patient (if a discharge note)

- Referral to other services; whether there are plans to consult with the patient's physician regarding further treatment or referral

An example follows:

> ### *E* X A M P L E
>
> **Intervention Plan:** Will be seen 3×/wk. as an outpatient. Will receive pulsed US to (R) anterior shoulder at 1.5 W/cm² for 5 min. followed by PROM & AROM exercises to (R) shoulder. Exercises will be followed c̄ an ice pack to (R) shoulder for 15 min. Pt. will be instructed in home exercise program for (R) shoulder AROM (attached).

The intervention plan portion of the note describes the plan for the patient's treatment *(what the patient will receive)*. This differs from describing the treatment and reaction to treatment mentioned in earlier parts of the note. If treatment or intervention is mentioned in earlier parts of the note, it may include specifics of *what was done with the patient that day and/or the patient's reaction to treatment.*

> ### *E* X A M P L E
>
> **O:** <u>Reaction to Rx:</u> Performed 10 reps each of quad sets & SLR to (L) LE; c̄ 10th repetition of SLR, Pt.'s quadriceps were fatigued & Pt. could no longer perform SLR.
> **P:** Cont. to see Pt. 1×/wk. to update home exercise program.

161

Relationship to Anticipated Goals

Once the anticipated goals are set, an intervention plan is then set up to achieve each of the anticipated goals. One exercise or intervention may achieve more than one anticipated goal. In fact, it is advantageous and economically sound to establish the intervention program to achieve the goals most efficiently. When setting up an intervention program, each anticipated goal, the patient's allotted time for therapy, the patient's endurance level, and the patient's level of boredom or interest must be considered.

E X A M P L E

Expected Outcomes:
1. Indep. walker amb. on level surfaces FWB for 70 ft. × 2 & 1 step within 10 days.
2. Indep. transfers sit ↔ stand & on/off toilet within 10 days.

Anticipated Goals:
1. Amb. c̄ walker 50% PWB Ⓡ LE for ~20 ft. × 2 within 5 days of Rx
2. Pt. will demonstrate transfers sit ↔ stand & on/off toilet c̄ min. assist + 1 within 5 days of Rx
3. Pt. will demonstrate Ⓡ quadriceps strength of @ least 2/5 within 5 days of Rx to assist. c̄ amb.
4. Pt. will be indep. in demonstrate exercises that he is perform in his room within 2 Rx sessions

Intervention Plan: BID in dept.: amb. training c̄ a walker beginning c̄ 50% PWB Ⓡ LE & progressing wt. bearing & distance as tolerated; transfer training; Pt. will be given written & verbal instruction in exercise program to be performed in his room (attached); AAROM progressing to AROM exercises Ⓡ knee emphasizing quadriceps functioning.

Writing the Intervention Plan

Here are some things to consider and include when writing the intervention plan.

Modalities:
  Which modality
  Where
  How long
  Intensity
  What position (one that is best, most comfortable)

Examples:
  US: W/cm², time, where, position, reaction, coupling agent
  Electrical stimulation: type of current, intensity, type of contraction, where, time, position
Ambulation:
  Distance
  Level of assistance
  Device(s)
  Time
  Weight-bearing status
  Type of gait pattern
Exercise:
  Extremity or trunk
  Types
  Repetitions
  Position
  Equipment used
  Modifications
  Amount of resistance given (or weight used)
  Home programs (usually attached to D/C notes as part of medical record):
    Brief goal/rationale statement
    Illustrations
    Position
    Directions: keep language simple and in patient terms
    Repetitions and times/day
    Progression
    Equipment
    Precautions

A Word About Interim Notes and Revision

The intervention plan needs to be revised as the patient's condition is reexamined and reevaluated new anticipated goals are set. When revision is necessary, the revision of the intervention plan is mentioned in an interim note, along with the changes noted during re-examination, re-evaluation, and the resetting of anticipated goals.

A Word About Discharge Notes

Generally, the following should be briefly stated:

• What interventions the patient received

• If instruction in a home program was done and how well the patient performed the home program

• If any other type of instruction was performed and the result of this instruction

- If the patient was sold any type of equipment (weights, assistive device, lumbar roll, and so on)

- If a referral to a home health agency or any other professional was made

If instruction of any kind is performed, the following information should be considered or recorded:

Who was instructed (patient, patient's family member)

The *type* of instruction (verbal, written, demonstration)

The level of the patient or patient's family functioning (could independently demonstrate, could correctly describe the activity, could state the precautions needed for ADL, and so on)

The discharge note should also include the following information:

- The number of times the patient was seen in therapy

- If and when the patient was not seen/on hold and why

- Any instances of the patient skipping or canceling treatment sessions

- To where the patient is discharged (rehabilitation center, skilled nursing facility, home)

- The reason for discharge from therapy (goals achieved, transfer to another facility or type of therapy, patient requested discharge from therapy, patient's death)

- Recommendations for follow-up treatment or care given to the patient

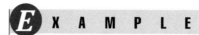

Intervention Plan: Pt. was seen BID for gait & transfer training & (L) LE AROM exercises (initial date) through (discharge date). Pt. refused Rx in P.M. of (date) and A.M. of (date) 2° severe nausea. D/C PT on this date p̄ 6 Rx sessions 2° D/C of Pt. from Hospital XYZ to home. Pt. & Pt.'s daughter were instructed in attached home program & given a copy of same program & Pt. was indep. in same program. A walker was ordered for Pt. per Pt. request. Pt. will be followed by ABC Home Health Agency for further therapy.

Summary

The Intervention Plan (P) part of the note is the final step in the planning process for patient care. In initial and interim notes, it outlines the interventions to be used with the patient. In discharge notes, it summarizes the interventions the patient received, the total number of intervention sessions, any patient education performed, handouts or equipment given or sold to the patient, and recommendations for future interventions or follow up care.

The worksheets that follow give you the chance to identify intervention plan statements and to write the intervention plan portion of the note. For the purposes of this workbook, you are not expected to generate an appropriate intervention plan without guidance. After reviewing the previous information, completing the worksheets, and comparing your work to the answer sheets, you should be able to write the intervention plan part of the note if you are given the information to be included.

Writing the Intervention Plan:

Worksheet 1

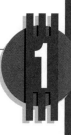

PART I. Mark the statements that should be placed in the Intervention Plan by placing an *IP* on the blank line before each statement. Also, mark the Expected Outcomes by marking *EO* on the line before the statement, and indicate Anticipated Goals by marking an *AG* on the line before the statement.

1. _____ Will be seen 3×/wk. as an OP.

2. _____ ↑ strength Ⓡ hip flexors, abductors and extensors to 3+/5 in 1 wk.

3. _____ Amb. training, working to ↑ wt. bearing Ⓡ LE & ↓gait deviations, progressing to uneven surfaces & obstacles.

4. _____ AROM exercises Ⓡ hip.

5. _____ ↑AROM Ⓡ hip to 100° flexion in 1 wk.

6. _____ Strengthening exercises Ⓡ hip musculature.

7. _____ Pt. will be able to amb. on level surfaces c̄ a straight cane s̄ gait deviations in 1 wk.

8. _____ Pt. will be instructed in home exercise program to ↑ strength Ⓡ hip musculature & ↑AROM Ⓡ hip

9. _____ Pt. will be able to stand on Ⓡ LE only for 10 seconds in 1 wk.

10. _____ Pt. will be able to amb. s̄ assist. device FWB for 300+ ft. × 2 indep. around obstacles & ↑ & ↓ stairs in order to participate in his normal community activities p̄ 3 wks. of OP Rx.

PART II. Write the following information into clear, concise statements regarding interventions (include verbs to make the phrases/sentences complete).

1. Hot pack—20 minutes—once per day—lumbar area

Answer: _____

_____

2. Continuous ultrasound—7 minutes—1.0 watts per centimeter squared—right upper trapezius muscle—three times per week

Answer: _____

_____

3. Twice per day—progress patient through knee exercise program—attached—bilat. knees

Answer: _____

_____

PART III. Read each of the following intervention plans and state what is missing.

1. Pt will receive compression pump Rx.

   Answer: _____

   _____

   _____

   _____

2. Pt. will receive whirlpool BID.

   Answer: _____

   _____

   _____

   _____

Answers to "Writing the Intervention Plan: Worksheet 1" are provided in Appendix A.

Writing the Intervention Plan:
Worksheet 2

PART I. Mark the statements that should be placed in the Intervention Plan by placing a *P* on the blank line before each statement. Also, mark the Expected Outcomes by marking *EO* on the line before the statement, and indicate Anticipated Goals by marking an *AG* on the line before the statement.

1. _____ Training in floor ↔ stand transfers.

2. _____ Pt. will be able to amb. FWB c̄ walker indep. on level surfaces for 5 blocks, stairs, & uneven surfaces to reintegrate Pt. into the community p̄ 4 wks. of Rx.

3. _____ Pt. will be given a home exercise program for general LE strengthening.

4. _____ Pt. will be able to perform floor ↔ standing indep. to ensure Pt's safety @ home & in the community within 4 wks. of Rx.

5. _____ Will be seen 3×/wk. in her home.

6. _____ Pt. will be able to perform sit ↔ stand transfers from a low chair in 1 wk. to prepare Pt. for floor ↔ stand transfers.

7. _____ Pt. will be able to amb. c̄ walker 500 ft. indep. in her home in 1 wk. to prepare Pt. for community amb.

8. _____ Pt. will ↑ LE strength to 4–/5 throughout bilat. within 1 wk. to improve amb. & floor ↔ stand transfers.

9. _____ Pt. will be able to amb. obstacles in her home c̄ walker indep. in 1 wk. to prepare Pt. for community amb.

10. _____ Amb. training FWB c̄ walker, beginning on level surfaces within the home & progressing to obstacles, stairs, & uneven surfaces.

11. _____ Pt. will be indep. in home exercise program within 1 wk. to assist. Pt. c̄ amb. & floor ↔ stand transfers.

PART II. Write the following information into the Intervention Plan part of the note.

1. Sue Smith will be seen three times per week as an outpatient. You will first give her a pulsed ultrasound to her right shoulder at 1.5 watts per cm^2 for seven minutes. She'll then get mobilization to her right shoulder. You'll end Rx c̄ an ice pack for 20 minutes. You also plan to teach her a home exercise program and attach a copy of it to your note. You also will seek an OT referral for an ADL evaluation because she states she cannot do anything for herself at home.

INTERVENTION PLAN: _____

_____

_____

_____

_____

_____

_____

2. Rodney Racecar will receive treatment twice per day. He will be taught proper care of his residual limb and how to wrap his residual limb. He will receive resistive range of motion exercises to his legs beginning with 10 repetitions each and increasing the number of repetitions to 3 sets of 30 repetitions. He will receive gait training with axillary crutches non–weight-bearing right leg and also transfer training sit to/from stand, on/off toilet, supine to/from sit.

INTERVENTION PLAN: _____

_____

_____

_____

_____

_____

_____

Answers to "Writing the Intervention Plan: Worksheet 2" are provided in Appendix A.

Final Review Worksheet:

Patient/Client Management Note: Examination, Evaluation, Plan of Care

SOAP Note: Problem, S, O, A, & P

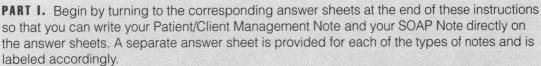

PART I. Begin by turning to the corresponding answer sheets at the end of these instructions so that you can write your Patient/Client Management Note and your SOAP Note directly on the answer sheets. A separate answer sheet is provided for each of the types of notes and is labeled accordingly.

  The following are the notes to yourself that you jotted down while reading the chart, interviewing the patient, and performing the objective tests. (While taking notes for yourself, you did not consult Hospital XYZ's approved abbreviations list nor were you particularly careful in your notation style.) Take some time to read through the information below before writing your notes.

 From the Chart

16 y.o. female
Pt. of Dr. Gungo
Fractured Right distal tibia and fractured right proximal humerus
ORIF Ⓡ proximal humerus on (date—yesterday)
Patient has a cast applied to the tibia and is in a sling for the fractured humerus

From the Interview

C/o pain in right ankle while in a dependent position (10 on a 0–10 pain scale) and severe
    pain (7 on a 0–10 pain scale) in right shoulder with elbow AAROM.
Lives c̄ parents—1 story house—1 step at entrance with no handrail—has carpeting through-
    out.
Never used a wheelchair before.
Patient is right handed.
Pt. was in a car accident with one friend—friend was driving—friend is OK and in the com-
    munity without injury at this time.
Is a high school student and wants to return to school ASAP p̄ D/C.
School is on one level with no steps to enter the school. However, distances between class-
    rooms are up to 1500 feet long. Has 7 class periods per day. All floor surfaces are
    linoleum.
School is very academically challenging and competitive and does not believe she can stay
    out of school until she is healed.
Parents attended therapy with patient; state their insurance will rent the patient a wheel-
    chair.
Patient and parents report patient is an athlete—on swim team at school—generally good
    health—swims daily all year.
No previous hospitalizations or serious illnesses.
Does not smoke cigarettes or drink ETOH.
Lives with both parents.
Pt.'s parents both work so Pt. will be @ home alone until she can go to school.

Pt. reports is having difficulty feeding herself and cannot dress herself. Has not seen OT.

Height: 5 ft. 6 inches, weight 125 pounds.

Pt. does not smoke or drink ETOH.

Family health history includes hypertension in both parents controlled by medication.

Patient is currently taking [pain medication]—takes no other medications regularly

X-ray revealed good alignment of Ⓡ LE fx in cast and good alignment of Ⓡ humerus after surgery.

Systems Review

(Some of this information is drawn from the chart and from the previous interview—see these sections to complete the systems review.)

Cardiopulmonary: not impaired

BP: 110/70

HR: 70

Resp. rate: 12

Edema: none noted

Integumentary: impaired

Disruption of skin at incision site right upper arm

Continuity of skin color—bruising Ⓡ UE and Ⓡ foot

Pliability—WNL Ⓛ extremities; Ⓡ extremities not tested this date

Musculoskeletal system—impaired

Gross symmetry—standing: cannot stand; sitting; WNL

Gross ROM: impaired Ⓡ UE & LE

Gross strength: impaired Ⓡ UE & LE

Neuromuscular system:

Gait: impaired

Locomotion: impaired

Balance: not impaired in sitting and cannot stand

Motor function: not impaired

Communication: age-appropriate—not impaired

Oriented × 3—not impaired

Learning barriers: none

Pt. best learns: listening as she tries an activity

Education needs: healing process; adaptation of home to w/c; w/c management, w/c propulsion; ADLs; safety c̄ w/c; home exercise program for Ⓡ UE

Tests and Measures Performed

Bruising noted all of Ⓡ UE and on toes of Ⓡ foot

Some bruising noted Ⓡ posterior trunk

Ⓛ UE—WNL AROM & strength

Ⓡ shoulder not examined due to fracture

Ⓡ elbow AAROM is 30–70°

Ⓡ hand and wrist AROM very slow but WNL when patient is encouraged to complete full ROM—verbal cues are definitely needed

Ⓡ biceps & triceps strength is 2/5

Musculature controlling the right wrist and hand strength is 3/5

Left LE—WNL AROM and strength

Right LE—WNL at knee and hip—AROM

Ⓡ LE—strength 5/5 at knee and hip

Ⓡ LE—short leg cast Ⓡ ankle and foot so not examined

Ⓡ LE—toes warm and normal color—able to wiggle toes

Toilet transfers not tested first visit

Sit to and from stand with maximal + 1 assist

Supine to and from sit with moderate assistance of one person

W/c to/from bed with maximal + 1 assist
NWB Ⓡ LE
NWB Ⓡ UE
Cried when Ⓡ ankle initially put in dependent position (pain level of 10)
Ⓡ ankle pain level subsided after Pt. put Ⓡ LE in a dependent position multiple times
Unable to manage Ⓡ wheelchair brakes, or leg rest
Propelled wheelchair 10 feet using left leg and arm and was too exhausted to continue;
　　required minimal assistance of 1 person and verbal cues to do so

 PART II. Write a Pt. management note using the pages provided to write the note.

Begin by writing about the examination. Don't forget to begin with the date you are writing the note. Write the History, Systems Review and Tests and Measures parts of the note.

Now write the Diagnosis part of the note. You believe that rigorous AROM to the right elbow, wrist, and hand are needed to prevent them from losing all strength and ROM. You also know that the patient's lack of mobility is due to her inability to use her right extremities due to her recent fractures. You also believe a referral to OT is essential to the Pt.'s rehab. process to assist her with eating, bathing, dressing, and managing items for return to school in a wheelchair. The patient's problems fall into Musculoskeletal Practice Pattern G: Impaired Joint Mobility, Muscle Performance and ROM Associated With Fracture.

Now write the Prognosis part of the note. You believe that the patient has excellent rehabilitation potential. You believe that the patient will be able to return home and to school with 2 weeks of rehabilitation. You believe that the patient cannot stay at home alone until he or she becomes independent in wheelchair propulsion & transfers. You also believe the patient will need assistance in moving the longer distances in the school (more than 500 feet).

Now write the Expected Outcomes part of the note. You believe all of these expected outcomes will be achieved by discharge in two weeks.

1. You will set the first expected outcome for transfers. You believe the patient will be independent in all of the transfers listed in the initial note. This will help the patient to be functional at home and at school. Write this information into expected outcome #1.
2. You will set the second expected outcome for wheelchair management. You believe the patient will be independent in wheelchair management (brakes and footrests) to be more functional at home and at school. Write this information into expected outcome #2.
3. You will set the third expected outcome for wheelchair propulsion. You judge that the patient will be independent in wheelchair propulsion for 500 feet twice in order to function at school. She will use her left UE and LE. Write this information into expected outcome #3.
4. You will set the fourth expected outcome for prevention of loss of function. You believe the patient will be able to prevent losing function in the right elbow, wrist, and fingers to maximize UE function when humerus is healed. Write this information into expected outcome #4.

Now set the anticipated goals.

1. Look at the first expected outcome. You think the patient will be able to transfer supine ↔ sit c̄ verbal cues by the end of 1 wk. Write this information into anticipated goal #1.
2. Continue to look at the first expected outcome. You think the patient will be able to transfer sit ↔ stand with minimal assistance of one person by the end of the first week of therapy. Write this information into anticipated goal #2.
3. Continue to look at the first expected outcome. You think the patient will be able to transfer w/c to and from the bed and on and off the toilet with moderate assistance of 1 person by the end of the first week. Write this information into anticipated goal #3.

4. Look at expected outcome 2. You believe the patient will be able to manage the brakes and footrests of the wheelchair using an extended brake lever on the right with verbal cues by the end of the first week of therapy. Write this information into anticipated goal #4.

5. Look at expected outcome 3. You believe the patient will be able to propel her wheelchair for approximately 100 feet by the end of the first week of therapy using her left arm and leg. Write this information into anticipated goal #5.

6. Look at expected outcome 4. You believe the patient be able to perform AROM to the right elbow, wrist, and fingers independently by the end of the first week. You believe the patient will be independent in performing a home program of AROM exercises to the right elbow, wrist, and fingers. Write this information into anticipated goal #6.

Now write the intervention plan for the patient.

You plan to see the patient BID at bedside. You plan to instruct the patient in transfers (list all of the transfers listed in anticipated goals #1 through 3). You plan to instruct the patient in wheelchair management (see wheelchair details in anticipated goal #4). You plan to instruct the patient in wheelchair propulsion. You plan to instruct the patient in a home exercise program for AROM to the right elbow, wrist, and fingers and give the patient a copy of the program. You plan on asking the patient to perform the program for you daily and to perform the program by herself in her hospital room twice a day. You have attached a copy of the home exercise program to this note.

Sign the note (remember to use the appropriate initials behind your name).

 PART III. Write a SOAP Note using the pages provided to write the note.

Begin by writing about the examination. Don't forget to begin with the date you are writing the note. Write the Problem, S, and O parts of the note.

Now write the A part of the note. Begin with the Diagnosis. You believe that rigorous AROM to the right elbow, wrist, and hand are needed to prevent them from losing all strength and ROM. You also know that the patient's lack of mobility is due to her inability to use her right extremities due to her recent fractures. You also believe a referral to OT is essential to the Pt.'s rehabilitation process to assist her with eating, bathing, dressing, and managing items for return to school from a wheelchair. The patient's problems fall into Musculoskeletal Practice Pattern G: Impaired Joint Mobility, Muscle Performance and ROM Associated With Fracture.

Now continue writing this part of the note by writing the Prognosis. You believe that the patient has excellent rehabilitation potential. You believe that the patient will be able to return home and to school with 2 weeks of rehab. You believe that the patient cannot stay at home alone until he or she becomes independent in wheelchair propulsion & transfers. You also believe the patient will need assistance in moving the longer distances in the school (more than 500 feet).

Now write the P, or Plan of Care, part of the note. Begin by writing the Expected Outcomes. These are to be achieved by the time of discharge, in 2 weeks.

1. You will set the first expected outcome for transfers. You believe the patient will be independent in all of the transfers listed in the initial note. This will help the patient to be functional at home and at school. Write this information into expected outcome #1.

2. You will set the second expected outcome for wheelchair management. You believe the patient will be independent in wheelchair management (brakes and foot rests) to be more functional at home and at school. Write this information into expected outcome #2.

3. You will set the third expected outcome for wheelchair propulsion. You judge that the patient will be independent in wheelchair propulsion for 500 feet twice to be more functional at school. Write this information into expected outcome #3.
4. You will set the fourth expected outcome for prevention of loss of function. You believe the patient will be able to prevent losing function in the right elbow, wrist, and fingers to maximize UE function when humerus is healed. Write this information into expected outcome #4.

Now continue the Plan of Care by setting the anticipated goals. These are to be achieved after one week of therapy.

1. Look at the first expected outcome. You think the patient will be able to transfer supine to and from sit with verbal cues by the end of 1 wk. Write this information into anticipated goal #1.
2. Continue to look at the first expected outcome. You think the patient will be able to transfer sit to and from stand with minimal assistance of one person by the end of the first week of therapy. Write this information into anticipated goal #2.
3. Continue to look at the first expected outcome. You think the patient will be able to transfer wheelchair to and from the mat and on and off the toilet with moderate assistance of 1 person by the end of the first week. Write this information into anticipated goal #3.
4. Look at expected outcome 2. You believe the patient will be able to manage the brakes and footrests of the wheelchair using an extended brake lever on the right with verbal cues by the end of the first week of therapy. Write this information into anticipated goal #4.
5. Look at expected outcome 3. You believe the patient will be able to propel her wheelchair for approximately 100 feet by the end of the first week of therapy using her left arm and leg. Write this information into anticipated goal #5.
6. Look at expected outcome 4. You believe the patient be able to perform AROM to the right elbow, wrist, and fingers independently by the end of the first week. You believe the patient will be independent in performing a home program of AROM exercises to the right elbow, wrist, and fingers. Write this information into anticipated goal #6.

Now complete the Plan of Care by writing the Intervention plan for the patient.

You plan to see the patient BID at bedside. You plan to instruct the patient in transfers (list all of the transfers listed in anticipated goals #1 through 3). You plan to instruct the patient in wheelchair management (see wheelchair details in anticipated goal #4). You plan to instruct the patient in wheelchair propulsion. You plan to instruct the patient in a home exercise program for AROM to the right elbow, wrist, and fingers and give the patient a copy of the program. You plan on asking the patient to perform the program for you daily and to perform the program by herself in her hospital room twice a day. You have a attached a copy of the home exercise program to this note.

Sign the note (remember to use the appropriate initials behind your name).

Patient/Client Management Note

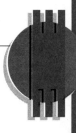

SOAP Note

Answers to "Final Review Worksheet" are provided in Appendix A.

PART V

Applications of Documentation Skills

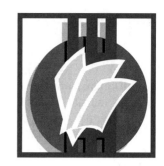

C ongratulations! You have mastered the skill of documenting patient care.
Now that you have mastered the skills involved in documentation, a brief discussion of applications of
documentation skills is needed. Applications of Note Writing and alternative formats to the Patient/Client
Management and SOAP note formats are presented (Chapter 16). Formulating alternatives to writing notes such
as documentation forms and computerized documentation are discussed (Chapter 17).

C H A P T E R

16 Applications and Variations in Note Writing

This workbook has covered the reasons for writing notes and a brief history of the origins of the two note formats. It has offered a test of your working knowledge of medical terminology and a good review of abbreviations.

As you begin to practice in clinical settings, you will find that nobody writes notes exactly as you were taught to write notes. Each facility that uses the Patient/Client Management Note or the SOAP Note format has its own variations of the format. Within any facility using a set note format, each therapist has his or her own variations of the format used by the facility.

Applying the Patient/Client Management & SOAP Notes to Other Note Formats

Many facilities do not use a Patient/Client Management or SOAP note format at all. Some facilities use a single narrative style format. Others use an outline format of some kind. Still others (especially private practice settings) may send letters to the patient's physician describing the patient's condition, goals, plans, and so forth. School settings and chronic care settings may set yearly goals as part of a student's or patient's individual education plan (IEP). Whatever format you may encounter, your knowledge of writing Patient/Client Management Notes and SOAP Notes should be helpful.

Narrative notes frequently include the same information used in the Patient/Client Management or SOAP note formats, but the information may be in a different order.

Outline note formats, or *fill-in-the-blank forms,* also include the information that the note formats in this book contain. The information may be organized in a different order, and periods or sentences

179

may not be used, but the information is still present. As long as you know how to organize the information and put the information into the categories used in the two note formats, you only need to learn where to put the information in an unfamiliar format or form.

Letters written to a physician's office on a regular basis are also usually organized in a particular style to save time. Certain categories are placed in a certain order, according to the standards set forth by the physical therapy practice involved. If you know the categories of the note formats taught in this workbook, you will be able to rearrange them to fit into a letter format.

IEPs also have a standardized format that takes the information involved in the note formats taught in this workbook and renames and rearranges the categories. Goals that are set yearly become the expected outcomes. Whether or not they are officially written, anticipated goals to be achieved by different times during the year are set to meet the expected outcomes. The goal format taught in this workbook is very adequate for use in most educational settings.

Finally, not every facility that writes SOAP Notes includes every part of the SOAP Note covered in this workbook. Many facilities include the expected outcomes and anticipated goals in the *A* part of the note. Others combine the *A* and *P* portions of the note and list each expected outcome, the corresponding anticipated goal(s), and interventions together before moving on to the next problem. There are as many variations on the SOAP Note as there are facilities that use the SOAP Note format.

Uses in Clinical Decision Making

One of the reasons that the note writing formats that you learned in this workbook are so adaptable to other styles of note writing is that they represent more than simple documentation formats. They represent a method of identifying, working through, and solving the patient's problems. Although you were not expected to independently identify the patient's diagnosis and prognosis, set expected outcomes or anticipated goals, or generate intervention plans in this workbook, you were given many examples of how the Patient/Client Management and SOAP note formats can be used to plan a patient's care. As long as you use the note formats for yourself in approaching and solving patient problems, you can learn to write the information in any form that you might like.

A Word to the PTA or COTA

Many of the examples in this workbook included writing an entire initial evaluation. According to the standards of the professions, PTAs and COTAs do not write initial notes. However, the skills that you used to write the initial notes in this workbook can be used in writing interim notes in your daily practice. Many facilities ask the assistant to write the interim note and to document the goals and interventions set by the therapist and assistant together for their patients. One of the ways in which you can be most helpful to the therapists with whom you work is to assist them with the documentation included in patient care. Therefore, it is important that your skills in this area continue to be used and improve long after you no longer need this workbook.

Documenting All Types of Patient Care

Most of the cases used in this workbook were very simple. Some of your instructors may disagree with the method of documenting the details of the cases listed within this workbook. (For example, there are quite a few acceptable methods of documenting AROM.) As you approach learning while in school and throughout your career, be aware of the methods available to document what you learn, no matter what the subject matter. Ask your instructors how they document the information that they are teaching you. Ask for definitions of terminology such as *minimal, moderate,* and *maximal* as you begin to practice in various clinical facilities. It is important that you keep abreast of research into therapy tests and measures and use the most reliable scales.

As professions, physical and occupational therapy have done much to standardize terminology used in documentation, but they still have much do to in this area. Many facilities do not have written definitions for commonly used terms, such as physical assistance given.

Your experience in writing notes and documenting what you do as a therapist has barely begun with the completion of this workbook. You have learned to write Patient/Client Management Notes and SOAP Notes, to organize the information into categories within each section of the note, to be clear and concise in what you say, and to use abbreviations and medical terminology well. The application of the information is now up to you.

As with any skill, the continued use and practice of note writing will perfect your skills. You will adapt all that you have learned about writing notes to the style of each facility in which you practice.

Eventually, even if you practice in a facility with a particular note-writing style, you will develop a style that is unique to you. You can develop expertise in documentation and help move the profession toward more standardized methods of evaluation and documentation.

In the immediate future, you may wish to remove the appendices from this workbook and keep them available as quick references on documentation. They summarize some of the information included in this workbook. They can assist you in applying what you have learned about writing notes as you continue the process of developing yourself as a member of the health-care team.

Alternatives: Documentation Forms, Medicare Forms, and Computerized Documentation

As trends in health care change, documentation changes. Health-care professionals are constantly looking for more efficient and effective ways to ease the task of documentation without losing their ability to act as professionals. Therefore, systems of documentation that can be performed at the point of care have been developed at some facilities and are currently being developed by other health care facilities and outside companies. In the meantime, Medicare has developed Forms 700 and 701 for purposes of obtaining consistent data that can assist Medicare reviewers with the determination of the appropriateness of the care given to patients.

Well-written Patient/Client Management Notes, SOAP Notes, documentation forms, Medicare forms, and computerized documentation share one characteristic: They provide structure to documentation. Structured documentation guarantees the collection of a consistent data set that can give us information about the outcomes and effectiveness of the interventions that we give our patients. Without this type of information, we will not be able to meet the challenges of managing both the cost and the quality of health care delivery.

▌ Medicare Forms

Medicare has developed Forms 700 and 701 in an attempt to gather consistent data needed to make decisions about whether the patient's condition and interventions qualify for Medicare coverage. Before these forms were developed, reviewers for Medicare were receiving poor-quality patient notes, some without goals, some without a good description of the patient's functional deficits. Medicare forms ask for (1) demographic information (the patient's name, age, and Social Security or Medicare number), (2) basic medical data (date of surgery or onset of condition, diagnosis), and (3) data that should already be contained in a well-written SOAP Note. The data they request include functional status prior to ther-

apy interventions and current functional status, long-term goals (expected outcomes), short-term goals (short-term goals, or anticipated goals, are listed as monthly goals), treatment (intervention) plan, and justification for treatment. It is easy to include the information required by these forms because the categories are similar to those of any good Patient/Client Management or SOAP note.

▌ Documentation Forms and Computerized Documentation Programs

In some facilities, forms are used for documentation or documentation is done on the computer. Facilities usually have unique documentation forms or some type of computerized documentation format. The purpose of this section is to review some advantages and disadvantages of each of these formats for documentation and to include items for consideration when developing forms or considering the purchase of a computerized documentation system.

Documentation Forms

Documentation forms are used in many clinics for many reasons. Some of the reasons include the following:

- Decreasing the amount of writing by the therapist/assistant
- Increasing the efficiency of the therapist/assistant in documenting patient care
- Increasing the consistency of documentation (and thus fulfilling certain quality assurance or legal/risk management requirements) by building certain components into a note, such as whether the patient is given a home program, and his or her level of independence in performing the home program

- Making the data gathered for outcomes studies more consistent
- Making functional information easier to read by all parties who use the information

Forms are usually individualized to fit the needs of the individual health care institution and its patient population. When designing a form, a good place to start is by watching clinicians practice. Forms should include the items commonly examined by the therapist. Other additions to the forms can be obtained by asking staff members to use the forms and give feedback to those designing the forms.

When beginning to use a new form, it is important for the therapist/assistant to give himself or herself time to adapt to the use of the form. Becoming familiar with the form before seeing a patient makes the therapist much more efficient in the use of the form.

The most efficient use of a form is to complete the form, or at least begin its completion, while seeing the patient. If you can write your examination findings directly on the form, you will save time. *Caution:* Do not let the use of forms limit your practice! If an item is missing from a form, find a place to write it (if it is relevant to the patient's function). Also, forms should be revised on a regular basis to meet the needs of good clinical practice.

Types of Documentation Forms

Several types of documentation forms are in use in various facilities. These include the following:

- Flow sheets
- Initial examination/discharge note forms
- Interim/discharge note forms
- One-visit-only documentation forms
- Supplement forms to be attached to initial, interim, or discharge forms (often have specialized tests or scales that are only needed with certain types of patients)

Development of Documentation Forms

When developing a form, the following should be considered:

- Do not reinvent the wheel unless you really must. Revising a form from another facility (used with permission, of course) is much easier than starting with nothing.
- When you have developed a draft version of the form, ask yourself and those who must use and read the forms if the form does what it is supposed to do for all parties involved (health-care providers, those concerned with reimbursement, and so on).
- Communicate with all parties involved when you develop forms. If the form is to be useful, everyone must know how to use the form (both writing on the form and reading the form).
- Examination items frequently used by the staff should be included.
- If a standard scale, test, or definition of measurement is used by all staff to measure or document a certain characteristic of the patient or a certain facet of patient care, a checklist may be faster in documenting the care.
- Checklists can save the therapist time and add speed in documentation.
- If you use any sort of checklists in your note forms, try to make the checklists consistent or similar from one form to another. This saves confusion and unnecessary staff reorientation time.
- Frequently leave space for very brief comments or descriptions.
- Unless the form is created with a very specific patient population in mind, allow for a general examination of the patient.
- If there are no standardized methods of documenting the information derived from your examination of the patient, allow room for writing.
- Forms influence practice, so make sure to include items that you believe are essential to practice.
- If the staff has been writing Patient/Client Management or SOAP notes, transition for the staff will be easier if you follow a format similar to SOAP or Patient/Client Management notes. Because these note formats are formats that support clinical decision-making, documentation using this format on a form assists the staff in clinical decision-making.
- Function should still be stated first in the examination portion of the note form, just as you should do so when writing notes.

Computerized Documentation

Computerized documentation continually changes and develops as technology improves. Some facilities have a well-developed program that is tailored to the needs of that facility. Within the next few years, many improvements will be seen in the area of computerized documentation. This section will serve as a review of some of the features that have been developed or are in stages of development by various companies and health-care systems throughout the country.

The advantage of computerized documentation over the use of forms is that the limitations of paper (trying to get all the necessary information into a limited amount of space) become unimportant because the computer is not limited to any particular size in which to place the information gathered. Computers can also have all of the possible tests and measurement available, so the therapist is not limited by the tests and measurements available on a given form.

Some features that will make computers even easier to use in the future are the following:

- *Data can be entered by making choices and simply touching a stylus to the screen or clicking a mouse.* This makes data entry more consistent and does not require keyboard competence.

- *Data can be printed in a variety of formats.* The Medicare Forms 700 and 701 no longer require extra time because the information can be printed in the format of a Form 700 or 701 for reimbursement purposes and in the format of a SOAP or Patient/Client Management note for the medical record. It could also allow the therapist to choose certain functional or relevant data to send to the patient's physician or other referral source.

- *The medical record can be retrieved and notes written at the patient's bedside.* Some health-care facilities have computers located in every patient's room or between every two rooms. With notebook and pocket-sized computer technology available, the therapist will be able to have a notebook with him or her that contains or can access the patient's medical record and rehabilitation information for all the patients the therapist treats.

- *All documentation can be completed at bedside.* Even outpatient and home health-care therapists will be able to have the computer with them and complete all documentation while they work with the patient. Notebook and pocket-sized computers with removable keyboards are already available. Modems make retrieval of the patient's medical record possible.

- *Handwriting recognition is a feature that has been developed and will continue to be developed in the next few years.* This will enable the therapist to enter extra notes and information as needed (much as therapists now do when they use forms and need to remark about the unusual quality of a movement).

- *Voice recognition is a feature that continues to be developed.* This could completely change our methods of data entry, although some caution must be taken in the use of voice-activated methodology while at the patient's bedside.

- *Charging will be able to be done by the therapist immediately upon completing the patient's care and while she or he completes other computerized documentation (and the computer may remind the therapist to charge the patient).* Computerized charging systems exist in many clinics today. Moving the charging to the patient's bedside, along with all other documentation functions, will greatly increase therapist efficiency and relieve the repetition in documentation that some therapists experience today.

When looking at computerized documentation systems, items that deserve consideration are listed in the following text:

- It is important to consider the needs of therapists at their individual practice sites. A system should be flexible enough to fulfill the needs of the therapist at the individual practice site; otherwise, the system is not worthwhile.

- Computerized documentation systems vary in their mobility, weight, flexibility, ease of use, speed of data entry, and speed of the hardware. All of these factors must be considered when purchasing or developing a computerized system.

- Training time must be taken into consideration when you discuss the cost of a computerized documentation system. A system that requires extensive training must also save much time to be cost effective.

- Technology is only worthwhile if it makes the therapist's task of documentation easier and allows her to do something he or she could not do without the technology. For example, the time spent documenting should be decreased, and spelling errors or obvious errors in recording of data should be pointed out to the therapist automatically for the purpose of immediate correction.

- The willingness, availability, and cost of programmers to customize the system to the individual facility's needs should be investigated before making a commitment to a computerized documentation system.

▌ Summary

Many facilities have found the development of documentation forms helpful in assisting therapists to document faster and more efficiently. Forms must be developed by a facility's therapists to meet their practice needs.

Computerized documentation will definitely be the mode of documentation in the future. Just as documentation forms must be customized to the practice at an individual practice site, computerized programs must be customized to meet the needs of therapists at an individual site.

Forms and computerized documentation do not exclude the type of thinking that is used in note writing. As mentioned previously, the Patient/Client Management and SOAP note formats assist therapists in structuring their thinking about patient problems and the attainment of the patient's goals for function. As forms and computer programs are further developed, aspects of clinical decision-making will continue to be used to assist the therapist in meeting patient needs while he or she documents.

Answers to Worksheets

Please note that you should not use Appendix A unless you have already completed the worksheets. Using these pages to initially complete the worksheets deprives the learner of the maximum benefit of this book.

C h a p t e r   3 :
Medical Terminology

● Worksheet 1

PART I

1. Osteoma
2. Hypoglycemia
3. Subcutaneous
4. Suprapubic
5. Dorsal/posterior
6. Cephalad
7. Erythema
8. Intercostal
9. Anterior or ventral
10. Afferent

PART II

1. Fusion of the pubic bones medially (growth of the bones together)
2. Enlargement of the heart
3. Removal of a meniscus
4. Cartilaginous tumor
5. Fusion of a joint
6. Surgical opening of the skull
7. The study of the nervous system
8. Without sensation
9. Inflammation of a vein
10. Abnormally high blood pressure

Medical Terminology

● Worksheet 2

PART I

1. Arthritis
2. Arthroscopy
3. Myopathy
4. Dyspnea
5. Ataxia
6. Chondromalacia
7. Encephalitis
8. Meningioma
9. Hemiplegia
10. Subclavicular

PART II

1. Without pain
2. Affecting both sides
3. Opposite side
4. Lack of speech
5. Inflammation of a tendon
6. Slowness of movement
7. Difficulty swallowing
8. Pain in the joints
9. Softening of the brain
10. Pertaining to a rib and its cartilage

C h a p t e r   4 :
Using Abbreviations

● Worksheet 1

1. The physician's orders say to do physical therapy in a wheelchair and turn the patient every hour.
2. In the chart it says the diagnosis is rheumatoid arthritis and rule out systemic lupus erythematosus.
3. Intervention Plan: OD, ADL training, US at 1.0 to 1.5 W/cm² to ant sup Ⓡ knee for 5 min.
4. Complains of shortness of breath after bilateral upper extremity proprioceptive neuromuscular facilitation exercises.
5. The medical diagnosis is multiple sclerosis and rule out organic brain syndrome.
6. Pt. is a B/K amputee. Hx of wearing PTB prosthesis c̄ a SACH foot for 20 yrs.
7. Pt. HR ↑ 20 BPM p̄ 2 min. of ADL.
8. Pt amb in // bars FWB Ⓛ LE ≈ 20 ft. × 2 c̄ min. assist. + 1. (or min. assist. of 1)
9. UE strength is 5/5 throughout bilat.
10. Anticipated Goal: ↓ dependence in transfers w/c → bed to mod. assist. within 1 wk.

Using Abbreviations

● Worksheet 2

1. The patient complains of right hip pain after ambulating 300 feet once with a walker full weight bearing right lower extremity.
2. Pt. may be 50% PWB Ⓛ LE.
   v.o. Dr. Smith/[your name], PT or OTR
3. Discontinue ultrasound in the area of the right sacroiliac joint.
4. The medical diagnosis is fractured left clavicle and subluxation of the left sternoclavicular joint.
5. Fasting blood sugar upon admission was over 300.
6. Medical dx: Ⓛ CVA.
7. Strength: 4/5 throughout UE bilat.

8. X-ray: fx (L) 3rd metacarpal proximal to MCP joint.
9. To OT for ADL.
   v.o. Dr. Jones/[your name], PT
Impression: peripheral neuropathy and rule out central nervous system dysfunction.

C h a p t e r 5 :
The Patient/Client Management Format: Writing History

● Worksheet 1

PART I

1.
2.
3. H
4.
5. H
6. H
7.
8.
9.
10. H
11.
12. H
13. H
14. H
15.

PART II

A. 10, 17, 14, 12, 22, 5
B. 3, 7, 27, 13, 15, 19
C. 20
D. 23, 24, 28, 26
E. 7, 30
F. 1
G. 21, 2
H. 29
I. 16
J. 8, 18, 9, 6, 11
K. 25
L. 4

PART III

1a. Demographics:
1b. Pt. is 83 y.o. African American E. Is (R)-handed.
2a. Current Condition:
2b. Pt. fell & hit (R) arm & head as she stood up from sofa.
3a. Other clinical tests:
3b. X-ray (R) UE was neg.
4a. Living Environment:
4b. Pt. lives in an assisted living apartment. Meals, laundry, & housekeeping services are provided. Assist c̄ bathing is available prn.
5a. Social Hx:
5b. Pt. stated health care is "unneeded & usually dangerous."

PART IV

Demographics: Pt. is 98 y.o. Caucasian ♀ referred by nursing staff & Dr. Frien. Social Hx: Pt's family provides emotional support. Pt. has beliefs about urinary incontinence that prevent her from discussing the problem with ♂ health-care professionals. Employment/Work: Until 1 mo. ago, Pt. was very active in recreational & social activities within the nursing home environment. Living Environment: Has used w/c past 10 days in the nursing home. States transfers in/out of w/c indep. but cannot propel w/c as far as the recreational therapy dept. Social/Health Habits: Pt. does not smoke or drink. Family Hx: htn. Medical/Surgical Hx: Includes htn. Has had difficulties c̄ bladder control for ~5 yrs. & incontinence has ↑ in past few wks. Hx of arthritis in knees for > 50 yrs. Current Condition(s)/Chief Complaint(s): States quit amb. 10 days ago 2° urinary incontinence c̄ standing. States does not know if she can amb. s̄ urinary incontinence. States keeps a towel in w/c to guard against problems with incontinence. Has not told the nurses & has not seen MD for urinary problem because "women are not supposed to talk with men about those things." Pt goals: to be able to amb. to recreational therapy dept. s̄ urinary incontinence problem. Functional Status/Activity Level: Pt. stopped amb. during past 2 wks. Currently refuses to amb. c̄ nursing staff. Denies arthritis as cause of refusing to amb. Medications: antihypertensive only. Other Clinical Tests: Urinalysis: normal 1 wk. ago.

Writing History

● Worksheet 2

PART I

A. 11, 1
B. 6
C. 7, 15, 10, 21, 25
D. 20, 9, 24
E. 23, 4, 18
F. 16, 2
G. 19, 26
H. 14, 8 or 8, 14
I. 22, 3
J. 5
K. 13, 17
L. 12

PART II

1.
2.
3.
4. H
5. H
6.
7. H
8.
9. H
10.
11. H

12.
13. H
14.
15.
16. H
17.
18. H
19.
20.

PART III

1. D
2. B
3. H
4. J or K
5. L
6. D or G
7. A
8. E
9. A or I
10. F
11. J
12. A
13. E
14. M
15. B
16. H
17. C
18. F
19. A
20. G
21. I
22. A
23. C
24. H
25. A
26. C
27. D
28. M
29. K

PART IV

Note: Use of brackets [ ] indicates that the statement could have been included in this section of the note or could be where it is listed elsewhere in the note.

HISTORY: Demographics: Pt. is 13 y.o. Caucasian female referred by Dr. Frume c̄ medical dx of subcapital fx Ⓡ hip. [Pt. is Ⓡ-handed.] Social Hx: Lives c̄ parents & 11 y.o. brother. Mother does not work outside the home & can assist Pt. upon D/C to home. School: Attends ABC Middle School in 7th grade; school has no steps. Living Environment: Lives in house c̄ carpeted floor surfaces except for kitchen. House has 3 steps to enter c̄ handrail Ⓡ ascending. General Health Status: Pt. & mother rate Pt.'s general health as excellent; no major life changes during past year. Social Health Habits: Denies hx of alcohol or tobacco use. Pt. is on volleyball team & practices volleyball daily. Family Hx: Pt.'s mother has hx of breast CA & Ⓡ mastectomy in 1997 c̄ no evidence of recurrence. Father has hx of Htn controlled by medication. Hx of heart disease

in maternal & paternal grandfathers. Development: Hx is WNL. Pt. is Ⓡ-handed. Pt. Medical/Surgical Hx: No previous injuries or hospitalizations. [No previous use of assistive devices.] Current condition: c/o "excruciating pain" in Ⓡ hip when moves Ⓡ LE. Pt. was playing volleyball & jumped & landed on Ⓡ hip. Functional Status: Pt. has not been out of bed. No previous use of assistive devices. Medications: Demerol for pain. Other Tests: X-ray shows subcapital fx Ⓡ hip c̄ pin in place. Hgb is 10.

C h a p t e r 6 : Systems Review

● Worksheet 1

PART I

1. SR
2. SR
3. Hx
4. Hx
5. SR
6.
7. SR
8. SR
9. Hx
10. SR
11. Hx
12. Hx
13. SR
14.
15. SR
16. SR
17.
18. Hx
19. SR
20. SR

PART II

1. E
2. C
3. C
4. B
5. E
6. D
7. B
8. A
9. A
10. D
11. C
12. C
13. C
14. E
15. E
16. B
17. A
18. E
19. D
20. E

PART III

SYSTEMS REVIEW: <u>Cardiovascular/Pulmonary System:</u> HR 92 bpm. BP: 130/83. RR: 30. <u>Integumentary System:</u> Skin integrity: multiple small tears in skin of bilat. UEs noted. Skin texture: thin & fragile. Skin color: multiple small hematomas noted below the skin. <u>Musculoskeletal System:</u> Gross AROM: impaired in (R) UE; otherwise WNL. Gross strength: impaired in (R) UE; otherwise WNL. Posture: impaired. Ht: 6 ft. 2 in. Wt: 180 lbs. Neuromuscular System: Gait: impaired. Locomotion: impaired. Balance: impaired. Communication: age-appropriate. Cognition: Oriented to person & place but not to date. Affect: Emotional/behavioral responses impaired when breathing is more difficult. <u>Learning Barriers:</u> requires hearing aid to be able to learn & communicate. <u>Learning Style:</u> best learns from demonstration followed by reminders in the form of pictures. <u>Education needs:</u> disease process, value of exercise, safety, use of adaptive equipment & assist. devices.

Systems Review

● Worksheet 2

PART I

1. Hx
2. SR
3. Hx
4. Hx
5. SR
6. Hx
7. SR
8. Hx
9. Hx
10. SR
12. Hx
13. Hx
14. Hx
15. SR
16. Hx
17. Hx

PART II

1. Cardiovascular/Pulmonary System
2. Cardiovascular/Pulmonary System
3. Musculoskeletal System
4. Musculoskeletal System
5. Musculoskeletal System
6. Integumentary System
7. Integumentary System
8. Neuromuscular System
9. Cardiovascular/Pulmonary System
10. Communication
11. Integumentary System
12. Musculoskeletal System
13. Integumentary System
14. Musculoskeletal System
15. Cognition

16. Education Needs
17. Neuromuscular System
18. Learning Style
19. Learning Style
20. Neuromuscular System
21. Affect
22. Cardiovascular/Pulmonary System

PART III

SYSTEMS REVIEW: <u>Cardiovascular/Pulmonary System:</u> Unimpaired. BP: 125/85. HR: 80 bpm. RR: 13 breaths/min. Edema (R) foot surrounding wound on plantar surface. <u>Integumentary System:</u> Impaired. Skin integrity: impaired. Wound noted plantar surface (R) foot. Skin color: red in area surrounding wound. Skin texture: thin & fragile on feet bilaterally. Scar tissue: none noted bilat. <u>Musculoskeletal System:</u> Gross symmetry: impaired LEs. Gross ROM: impaired bilat. feet & ankles. Gross strength: impaired bilat. LEs. Ht: 6 ft. 2 in. Wt: 190 lbs. <u>Neuromuscular System:</u> Locomotion: unimpaired. Gait: impaired. Balance: impaired. <u>Communication:</u> unimpaired. <u>Cognition:</u> orientation unimpaired. <u>Affect:</u> emotional/behavior responses unimpaired. <u>Learning Barriers:</u> Sight impaired 2° cataracts; does not wear glasses. <u>Learning Style:</u> Learns best by demonstration by therapists accompanied by HEP that includes illustrations. <u>Education Needs:</u> disease process, safety, wound care, exercise program, ADLs, use of assist. device, general foot care, appropriate foot wear.

Chapter 7:
Tests and Measures

● Worksheet 1

PART I

1. TM
2. H
3.
4.
5.
6. TM
7. Sr
8. H
9. TM
10. H
11.
12. TM
13. TM
14. H
15. TM
16.
17.
18. TM
19.
20. H

PARTS II and III

1. D
   Impair
2. B
   Func
3. E
   Impair
4. D
   Impair
5. E
   Impair
6. E
   Impair
7. C
   Impair
8. E
   Impair
9. E
   Impair
10. A
    Func
11. D
    Impair
12. E
    Impair
13. B
    Func
14. D
    Impair
15. E
    Impair

PART IV

Headings should be the following:
Transfers
Amb
Activity Tolerance
Strength
AROM

PART V

A. 2
B. 1
C. 4, 3 (any order of these two statements is OK)
D. 5
E. 6

PART VI

Amb: Pt. stood in // bars c̄ min. + 1 assist. FWB bilat. LEs × 2. Transfers: sit ↔ stand c̄ min. + 1 assist. Strength: UE & LE strength @ least 3/5 (group muscle test); unable to further examine due to Pt.'s mental status. ROM: UE & LE WNL except ~90° shoulder abduction & ~110° shoulder flexion bilat. Activity tolerance: fatigued p̄ standing × 2; all other examination deferred.

Tests and Measures

● Worksheet 2

PART I

A. 3, 7
B. 5, 4, 1, 2
C. 6

PART II

There are probably many correct ways to organize this information. This student did a nice job organizing the information. Another way to organize it would be to use the following categories: Amb, Transfers, Ⓡ UE, Ⓛ UE & LEs. This method would allow the reader to see that the Ⓛ UE and LEs are relatively normal and then to get an accurate view of the Ⓡ UE.

TESTS & MEASURES: Amb.: c̄ walker c̄ min + 1 assist. for 50 ft. × 1 wt. bearing as tolerated all extremities. Transfers: W/c ↔ mat pivot c̄ min + 1 assist. (or + 1 min. assist. or c̄ min. assist. of 1), sit ↔ supine indep. Ⓡ UE: *Appearance:* Incision Ⓡ ant. forearm covered c̄ steristrips. *AROM:* Limited shoulder flex. To ~120°, abd. To 70°; elbow flex. WNL, ext. –42°; wrist flex. WNL, ext. to neutral c̄ full finger flex. *Strength:* Ⓡ shoulder flex. 3+/5; elbow flex. & ext., wrist flex & ext, wrist flex & ext, fingers flex & ext 4/5. *Sensation:* WNL to light touch & sharp/dull. Ⓛ UE & LEs: *AROM:* WNL throughout. *Strength* (gross break test used): 5/5 throughout Ⓛ UE & Ⓡ LE. Ⓛ LE 4/5 all muscle groups. *Sensation:* To light touch & sharp/dull WNL throughout.

Review Worksheet: Writing the History, Systems Review, and Tests and Measures

PART I

1. TM
2.
3.
4. Hx
5. TM
6. Hx
7. Hx
8. Hx
9. TM
10. Hx
11. TM
12. TM
13. Hx
14.
15.

PART II

1a. Hx
1b. Current Condition/chief complaint
1c. C/o intermittent Ⓛ lat. knee pain
2a. Tests and Measures

2b. Sensation
2c. ↓ sensation Ⓛ L5 dermatome
3a. Hx
3b. Other tests
3c. Arthroscopy on 02/02/2002
4a. Hx
4b. Current condition
4c. Craniotomy Feb. 2002
5a. Tests & Measures
5b. PROM
5c. Ⓡ LE PROM is WNL throughout.

PART III

Information in brackets [ ] could go in this category instead of the one in which it was placed.

01/14/2002. HISTORY. Demographic Info.: Pt. is a 65 y.o male patient referred by Dr. Sosome. Medical Dx: fx Ⓡ femoral neck on 01/12/2002. Ⓡ hip prosthesis insertion on 01/13/2002. PT [OT] attempted to see Pt. on 01/14/2002; examination deferred due to low HgB & Pt. dizziness while supine. Current condition: c/o pain Ⓡ hip 8/10 standing & 4/10 supine (prior to amb.). Pt. fell at home & hit Ⓡ hip on bathtub, causing fx. Currently seeing OT for dressing & grooming issues. Pt. goals: to amb. indep. s̄ device (long term). [OT: Would like to be indep in grooming and dressing & would "settle" for Meals on Wheels.] Would like to return to her apartment @ D/C (short term). Functional status/activity level: States has had no PT or OT PTA. Has never used an assist. device PTA. Owns no assist. devices for dressing, grooming, bathing, toileting or amb. PTA watched her toddler-aged grandchildren 1×/wk. & played cards c̄ friends 2 noc/wk. Volunteers @ elementary school 3 days/wk, reading c̄ children. Social hx: Lives alone. Living environment: Lives in a senior apartment building. Has an elevator; has to amb. curbs only. Apartment bathroom has a bathtub c̄ a shower & shower curtain. Employment status: Retired in past yr. [Volunteers @ elementary school 3 days/wk., reading c̄ children.] Social/health habits: denies ETOH & drug use. Walks ~2 mi. 3×/wk. [Medical/surgical hx: fx Ⓡ femoral neck on 01/12/2002. Ⓡ hip prosthesis insertion on 01/13/2002. PT [OT] attempted to see Pt. on 01/14/2002; examination deferred due to low HgB & Pt. dizziness while supine.] Other clinical tests: HgB 7 on 01/14/2002. Blood transfusion on 01/14/2002. HbG 11 on this date.

SYSTEMS REVIEW. Cardiopulmonary: unimpaired. BP: 140/80. HR: 80. Resp. rate: 12. Integumentary: impaired at surgery site; otherwise unimpaired. Musculoskeletal: Gross strength impaired Ⓡ LE. Gross ROM impaired Ⓡ LE. Neuromuscular system: gait impaired, locomotion impaired, balance impaired in standing & during amb., motor function impaired. Communication: unimpaired. Affect: emotional/behavioral responses unimpaired. Cognition: oriented × 3. Unimpaired. Learning barriers: wears glasses & cannot read s̄ them; will need glasses to learn home exercise program. Learning style: visual learner; prefers to watch & then imitate PT's actions. Education needs: ambulation training & safety c̄ walker on level surfaces & curbs, transfer training & safety, info. on proper progression & healing of incision site, home exercise program

TESTS & MEASURES (PT). Transfers: w/c ↔ bed & supine ↔ sit c̄ mod. + 1 assist. Sit ↔ stand c̄ min. + 1 assist. Amb.: // ~20 ft. × 1 50% PWB Ⓡ LE c̄ min. + 1 assist. Pt. became dizzy & nauseated p̄ amb. & examination terminated p̄ exam. UEs & Ⓛ LE: Strength 4+/5 throughout. ROM: WNL except –5° Ⓡ elbow ext. Ⓡ LE: ROM: limited 2° post-op restrictions to 90° hip flex, full active hip abduction, 0° hip medial & lateral rotation, 0° abduction. Strength: @ least 3/5 throughout; not further examined 2° recent surgery. Exercise tolerance: BP: 145/90 p̄ amb., 135/80 3 min. p̄ amb. HR: 105 p̄ amb., 82 3 min. p̄ amb. Resp Rate: 18 p̄ amb., 12 3 min. p̄ amb.

TESTS & MEASURES (OT). Pt. initially seen B/S for examination of grooming & dressing skills. Bathing: Able to bathe UEs & truck c̄ supervision & setup of sponge bath; requires min. + 1 assist. to bathe LEs. Grooming: Grooms hair indep. Dental care indep. Contact lens management indep. Dressing: not tested this date 2° high pain level & ↓ Pt. endurance. Transfers: supine ↔ sit & w/c ↔ bed c̄ mod. assist. of 1. UEs: Strength 4+/5 per group muscle test. AROM: WNL except –5° Ⓡ elbow ext. Fine motor skills WNL.

C h a p t e r   9 :
Subjective

● Worksheet 1

PART I

1. S
2.
3. [This is *not* S because objective testing is required to ascertain whether the motion reproduces the pain.]
4.
5.
6. S
7.
8.
9. S
10. Prob
11.
12.
13.
14. S
15.
16. Prob
17.
18.
19.
20. S
21.
22. S

PART II

1. Dx: Ⓡ shoulder bursitis.
2. Problem: 75 y.o. Caucasian male c̄ dx of Ⓛ shoulder subluxation. S/p Ⓡ stroke ~1 yr.
3. Dx: respiratory failure. Hx: COPD, CHF, Htn

PART III

A. 1, 4, 6, 2, 12
B. 10, 7
C. 3
D. 5, 9, 18, 20
E. 8, 13
F. 14
G. 3, 15, 17, 19, 21
H. 16
I. 11

PART IV

1a. Current condition:
1b. Pt. fell in her living room.
1c. (1) When did the patient fall?
    (2) How did the patient fall?
    (3) What was the patient doing when she fell?
2a. Current condition:
2b. States onset of pain in the P.M. of [date].
3a. Current condition:
3b. C/o min. pain (R) foot on this date.
3c. (1) The exact location of the pain in the (R) foot.
    (2) Rating the pain on a pain scale.
4a. Living environment:
4b. States lives alone. Describes 2 steps c̄ handrail on (R) ascending @ entrance of her home.
5a. Current condition:
5b. States pain radiates from (R) hand through (R) forearm on this date, limiting typing to 5 min. ā requires rest.

PART V

Problem: 58 y.o. ♂ referred from E.D. by Dr. Sleet. Medical dx: minor ligamentous injury (R) knee. X-ray (R) knee neg.

  S: Current Condition: c/o constant, "burning" (R) knee pain; rates pain as 7 (0 = no pain, 10 = worst possible pain). Pain ↓ c̄ rest & ↑ c̄ walking. Denies pain while bending (R) knee. Fell @ work & landed on (R) knee. Functional status: Denies previous use of crutches. States can borrow crutches from a co-worker. Employment status: States is a carpenter; is on his feet most of the work day. Social history: Lives c̄ wife; wife works & is not available to assist. Pt. during the day. Living environment: Lives in apartment on 2nd floor c̄ 9 steps to enter c̄ handrail on the (L) ascending. No elevator is available. General health status: States general health good; gets lots of exercise each day @ work. Does not smoke. Medical/Surgical History: No significant history of disease, serious illness, or injury. History of spring allergies. Medications: Takes [prescription allergy medication]. Family health history: Htn in 2/5 siblings & both parents. Patient goals: Short term: to be able to access apartment indep. Long term: to resume former busy lifestyle, including returning to work asap.

  Interim note follows:
  S: Current condition: c/o pain c̄ typing; rates pain as 5 (0 = no pain, 10 = worst pain). Pain ↓ c̄ rest & ↑ c̄ grasping or wt. bearing activities (L) UE. Fell @ work [date] & landed on (L) hand c̄ wrist extended so pain has ↑ since last seen by PT on [date]. X-rays of (L) wrist & hand @ physi-

cian's office p̄ fall were neg. Also c/o edema & stiffness (L) hand & wrist c̄ active movement. Edema is ↑ p̄ work. Functional activities: is having difficulty eating c̄ (R) hand; is (L) hand dominant. Employment: Pt. types @ work up to 8 hrs./day. States physician told him to limit types to 4 hrs./day until edema stops. New Pt. goal: to be able to hold a fork s̄ pain (short term).

Subjective

● Worksheet 2

PART I

A. 9, 1
B. 3, 5
C. 7
D. 10, 2
E. 6, 8
F. 4
G. 11

PART II

1a. Current condition
1b. C/o pain (R) LE proximal to the knee.
1c. (1) Exact location of the pain is still unclear. Is the pain in the anterior or posterior portion of the (R) LE proximal to the knee?
    (2) Putting the pain on a pain scale would have been helpful.
2a. Functional status/social history (either answer would be correct)
2b. States depended on his wife to bathe him prior to this stroke. Plans to cont. to depend on wife for bathing p̄ D/C.
3a. Functional activities
3b. States cannot dress herself.
4a. Functional activities
4b. Denies use of a walker PTA.

PART III

1.
2.
3.
4. S
5.
6.
7. S
8.
9.
10. Prob
11. S
12.
13.
14.
15. S
16.
17.
18.
19. S

PART IV

Problem: Medical dx: Contusion (L) hip.

S: <u>Current condition:</u> C/o (L) hip pain when FWB (L) LE; pain intensity is 8 (0 = no pain; 10 = worst possible pain). Denies pain when in sitting or supine position. Fell on (L) hip at home in morning; was able to get up s̄ help. States experienced pain throughout day & went to ED in late P.M. <u>Functional ability:</u> Amb. indep. s̄ assist. device & all ADL tasks prior to injury. Currently spends time in a w/c rented by the family. <u>Living environment:</u> Lives alone in apartment c̄ an elevator. Needs to amb. curbs only. <u>Social history:</u> types bulletin & helps clean @ her church on a volunteer basis. <u>Medical history:</u> unremarkable except total hip replacement (L) in 1990. Used a walker @ that time. No history of hospitalization except for child-bearing. Does not take medications.

C h a p t e r   1 0 :
Objective

● Worksheet 1

PART I

1.
2. O
3.
4. S
5. O
6. S
7.
8. S
9. Prob
10. O
11.
12. O
13. S
14.
15. S
16.
17.
18.
19. O
20. O
21.
22. S
23.

PART II

1. E
2. F
3. E
4. A
5. B
6. F
7. A
8. D
9. G
10. C

11. B
12. F
13. A
14. C

PART III

1a. Strength
1b. Pt. has 4/4 strength in bilateral UEs.
2a. Trunk
2b. SLR (L) LE reproduces Pt.'s worst back pain.
3a. Strength
3b. 5/5 (R) shoulder musculature, 4/5 R biceps, 2/5 (R) triceps, 0/5 (R) UE musculature distal to elbow. (L) UE is 5/5.
4a. Amb.
4b. Pt. amb. ~150 ft. FWB c̄ walker ×2 indep.
5a. Reaction to Rx:
5b. Pt. was SOB p̄ transfers supine ↔ sit and bed ↔ B/S chair; resp. rate ↑ from 18 breaths/min. ā transfer to 32 breaths/min. immediately p̄ the transfer.
6a. AROM
6b. (L) ankle is WNL.

PART IV

1. Cardiovascular unimpaired. BP: 110/65. HR: 75 bpm. Resp. rate 14
2. Integumentary unimpaired.
3. Musculoskeletal: impaired (R) LE.
4. Neuromuscular: impaired gait & locomotion; motor function unimpaired; balance impaired.
5. Communication: age appropriate & unimpaired.
6. Affect: unimpaired.
7. Cognition: unimpaired; oriented × 3.
8. Learning barriers: none noted.
9. Learning style: visual; prefers demonstration prior to attempting movement.
10. Educational needs: amb. c̄ walker & walker safety; transfer safety; protection of cast
11. <u>Bilat UEs:</u> Strength & AROM WNL.
12. <u>Amb.:</u> indep. c̄ walker NWB LE 50 ft. × 2.
13. (L) LE: long leg cast applied.
14. (R) LE: AROM WNL. Strength 5/5 throughout.
15. <u>Transfers:</u> on/off toilet c̄ min. + 1 assist. Sit ↔ stand & supine ↔ sit indep.
16. <u>Amb.:</u> ↑ & ↓ 1 step c̄ walker c̄ min. + 1 assist.
17. <u>Amb.:</u> in & out of door, including opening & closing door, c̄ walker c̄ min. + 1 assist.
18. (L) LE: Not examined further this date.

PART V

A. 1, 2, 3, 4, 5, 6, 7, 8, 9, 10
B. 12, 17, 16
C. 15
D. 11, 14
E. 13, 18

PART VI

O: SYSTEMS REVIEW: <u>Cardiovascular:</u> unimpaired. BP: 110/65. HR: 75 bpm. Resp. rate 14. <u>Integumentary:</u>

unimpaired. <u>Musculoskeletal:</u> impaired Ⓡ LE. <u>Neuromuscular:</u> impaired gait & locomotion; motor function unimpaired; balance impaired. <u>Communication:</u> age appropriate & unimpaired. <u>Affect:</u> unimpaired. <u>Cognition:</u> unimpaired; oriented × 3. <u>Learning barriers:</u> none noted. <u>Learning style:</u> visual; prefers demonstration prior to attempting movement. <u>Educational needs:</u> amb. c̄ walker & walker safety; transfer safety; protection of cast. AMB: Indep. c̄ walker NWB Ⓛ LE 50 ft. × 2. Amb. ↑ & ↓ 1 step & in/out of door, including opening & closing door, c̄ walker NWB Ⓛ LE c̄ min. + 1 assist. TRANSFERS: On/off toilet c̄ min. + 1 assist. Sit ↔ stand & supine ↔ sit indep. UEs & Ⓡ LE: Strength & AROM WNL throughout. Ⓡ LE: long let cast applied. Not examined further this date.

Objective

● Worksheet 2

PART I

A. 6
B. 1
C. 2
E. 7, 4, 3, 5

PART II

O: W/C PROPULSION & MANAGEMENT: Propels w/c indep. 15 ft. × 1. Has difficulty parking w/c close to mat & locking brakes. Requires max + 1 assist to remove armrest. TRANSFERS: W/c ↔ mat c̄ sliding board NWB Ⓡ LE c̄ min + 1 assist. & verbal cues for hand placement; requires max + 1 assist. to place sliding board. Sit ↔ supine c̄ mod. + 1 assist to move Ⓡ LE. LE STRENGTH: Hip flexors: 4/5 Ⓛ, 3–/5 Ⓡ. Hip extensors: 4/5 Ⓛ, 3/5 Ⓡ. Hip abduction bilat. at least 3/5; not tested c̄ resistance against gravity. Knee flexors: 4/5 Ⓛ; 2–/5 Ⓡ. Knee extensors: 4/5 Ⓛ; 3/5 Ⓡ. Ankle 5/5 bilat. all movements. REACTION TO RX: Performed Ⓡ & Ⓛ hip abd/add. c̄ 2# × 15 (supine); knee flex. c̄ 2# × 15 Ⓛ, 1# × 15 Ⓡ; Ⓛ & Ⓡ terminal knee ext. c̄ 2# × 15. Requires frequent rests.

PART III

1a. Ambulation or gait
1b. Amb. c̄ walker 50% PWB Ⓛ LE for 50 ft. × 2 c̄ SBA to compensate for vision deficits.
2a. Systems review; cardiopulmonary subsection.
2b. Pitting edema Ⓛ LE noted.
3a. Reflexes
3b. KJ: 3+ Ⓡ, 2+ Ⓛ
4a. Transfers
4b. Transfers w/c ↔ mat c̄ min. assist. of 1 to stabilize balance loss.
5a. Rolling or bed mobility
5b. Requires max assist. of 2 to roll supine → Ⓡ or Ⓛ.
6a. Systems Review, Learning Barriers Subsection
6b. No learning barriers noted.

Review Worksheet: Stating the Problem, S, and O

PART I

1. O
2.
3.
4. S
5. O
6. Prob
7. S
8. S
9. O
10. Prob
11. O
12. O
13. S
14.
15.

PART II

1a. Subjective, or S
1b. Current condition
1c. C/o intermittent Ⓛ lat. knee pain
2a. Objective, or O
2b. Sensation
2c. ↓ sensation Ⓛ L5 dermatome.
3a. Subjective, or S
3b. Current condition
3c. States had an arthroscopy on 02/02/2002.
4a. Subjective, or S
4b. Current condition
4c. States had craniotomy in Feb. 2002
5a. Objective, or O
5b. Ⓡ LE or PROM or ROM
5c. Ⓡ LE PROM is WNL throughout

PART III

01/15/2002: Problem: Dx: Fx Ⓡ femoral neck 01/12/2002. Ⓡ hip prosthesis inserted 01/14/2002. HgB 7 on 01/15/2002. HgB 11 on this date.

S: <u>Current condition:</u> c/o pain Ⓡ 8/10 (0 = no pain, 10 = worst possible pain) while standing & 4/10 supine (prior to amb.). States fell @ home & Ⓡ hip it side of bathtub. <u>Living environment:</u> Lives in senior apartment building c̄ elevator; needs to amb. curbs only to enter. Apartment bathroom has bathtub c̄ shower & shower curtain. Has had no PT or OT services PTA. No walker or cane use PTA. Owns no assist. devices for bathing, toileting, dressing, or amb. <u>Social hx:</u> Lives alone. <u>Employment hx:</u> Retired in past yr. Volunteers @ elementary school 3 days/wk., reading c̄ children. <u>Functional status/activity level:</u> For recreation, Pt. plays cards c̄ friends 2 nocs/wk. & watches toddler-aged grandchildren 1×/wk. Social/health habits: Does not smoke or drink. Walks ~2 mi. 3×/wk. <u>Pt. goals:</u> Would like to return to her apartment p̄ D/C. (PT:) Would like to amb. indep s̄ device (long term). (OT:) Would like to indep. in grooming & dressing herself; would accept Meals on Wheels.

O: SYSTEMS REVIEW: <u>Cardiopulmonary</u>: unimpaired. BP: 140/80. HR: 80. Resp. rate: 12. <u>Neuromuscular</u>: gait, locomotion, balance in standing & during amb., & motor function impaired. <u>Integumentary</u>: impaired at surgery site; otherwise unimpaired. <u>Musculoskeletal</u>: ROM & gross strength impaired on Ⓡ LE. <u>Communication</u>: unimpaired. <u>Affect</u>: emotional/behavioral responses unimpaired. <u>Cognition</u>: oriented × 3, unimpaired. <u>Learning barriers</u>: wears glasses & cannot read s̄ them; will need glass for home exercise program. <u>Learning style</u>: visual learner; prefers watching therapist & then imitating actions of therapist. <u>Educational needs</u>: use of walker on level surfaces & curbs & safety c̄ walker, transfer training & safety, proper healing & monitoring of incision site, home exercise program. TRANSFERS: w/c ↔ bed & supine ↔ sit c̄ moderate assist. of 1 person. Sit ↔ stand c̄ min assist. of 1 person. AMB: // bars min. assist. of 1 person ~20 ft. ×1 PWB Ⓡ LE; Pt. then felt dizzy & nauseated so PT session was terminated @ that time. UEs & Ⓛ LE: ROMs WNL throughout except −5° Ⓡ elbow extension. Strength 4+/5 throughout (group muscle test). Ⓡ LE: ROM limited 2° post-op restrictions to 90° hip flex, full hip abduction AROM, 0° hip medial & lateral rotation, 0° adduction. Strength: @ least 3/5 throughout; not examined further 2° recent surgery. EXERCISE TOLERANCE: BP 145/90 p̄ amb, 135/80 3 min. p̄ amb. HR: 105 p̄ amb, 82 3 min. p̄ amb. Resp. rate: 18 p̄ amb, 12 3 min. p̄ amb.

[For the OT, beginning c̄ the section on transfers:]

TRANSFERS: w/c ↔ bed & supine ↔ sit c̄ mod + 1 assist. BATHING: Able to bathe trunk & arms c̄ supervision & setup of sponge bath; bathes LEs c̄ min. + 1 assist. GROOMING: Grooms hair indep. Dental care indep. Indep. management of contact lenses from w/c. DRESSING: not tested this date 2° ↑ pain level & ↓ Pt. endurance. UEs: Strength 4+/5 throughout (group muscle test). AROMs WNL except −5° Ⓡ elbow extension. Fine motor skills WNL.

Chapters 11 & 12

● Worksheet 1

PART I

1. T & M
2. Systems Review
3. H
4. H
5. H
6.
7. Diag.
8.
9. Prog.
10. H
11. H
12. H
13. Prog.
14. T & M
15. Systems Review
16.
17. H
18. Prog.
19. Diag.
20. Prog.
21. H
22. T & M

PART II

1. Diag.
2. Prog.
3. Prog.
4. Diag.
5. Prog.

PART III

1. DIAGNOSIS: Gait deviations & need for assist. in amb. c̄ an assist. device prevent Pt. from functioning at home indep. & from doing her work as a cashier outside of the home. Inability to use Ⓛ UE in a functional manner is affecting Pt.'s ability to perform ADLs. <u>Practice Patterns</u>: 1°Neuromuscular D: Impaired Motor Function & Sensory Integrity Associated c̄ Nonprogressive Disorders of the CNS—Acquired in Adolescence or Adulthood. 2° Musculoskeletal G: Impaired Joint Mobility, Muscle Performance, & ROM Associated c̄ Fx. Neuromuscular Pattern is 1° due to greater extent of deficits involved. PROGNOSIS: Pt. has good rehabilitation potential. Pt. is relatively young, motivated, cooperative & cognitively sound.

2. DIAGNOSIS: ↓ function in transfers is impairing Pt.'s ability to participate in activities in nursing home and is placing the health of nursing home staff at risk. <u>Practice Pattern</u>: Musculoskeletal J: Impaired Joint Mobility, Motor Function, Muscle Performance & ROM Associated c̄ Amputation. PROGNOSIS: Rehabilitation potential is fair because of Pt.'s medical dx of Alzheimer's Disease. Pt. follows simple commands & should be able to learn to transfer bed ↔ w/c c̄ min. assist. of 1 & verbal cues. This would ↓ risk and burden to caretakers, maximize activity level & quality of life, & prevent further pulmonary & integumentary problems.

● Worksheet 2

PART I

1. S
2.
3. O
4. O
5. O
6.
7. Diag.
8. S
9. Prob.
10. O
11. Diag.
12. O
13. S

14. Prog.
15. Prog.
16. O
17. O
18. Diag.
19. O
20. Prog.

PART II

1. Prog.
2. Diag.
3. Diag.
4. Prog.
5. Diag.

PART III

1. DIAGNOSIS: Pt.'s ↓ ROM & strength Ⓡ wrist cause
   Pt. difficulty in ADLS such as eating & writing. Pt.'s
   work involves typing over 50% of the time & Pt. is
   unable to type s̄ pain. Practice Pattern:
   Musculoskeletal G: Impaired Joint Mobility, Muscle
   Performance, & ROM Associated c̄ Fx.
   PROGNOSIS: Pt. has good rehab. potential; should
   progress well with PT.
2. DIAGNOSIS: Pt.'s Ⓡ extremity strength, motor plan-
   ning & mobility impairments will prevent the Pt. from
   returning home alone. Will need to regain indep. amb.
   & ADLs to return home. Practice Pattern:
   Neuromuscular D: Impaired Motor Function &
   Sensory Integrity Associated c̄ Nonprogressive
   Disorders of the CNS—Acquired in Adolescence or
   Adulthood.
   PROGNOSIS: Rehab. potential is fair. Pt. may need
   prolonged time to regain movement of Ⓛ extremities
   & overall mobility due to her advanced age.

Review Worksheet:
History, Systems Review, Tests &
Measures, Diagnosis, Prognosis
Problem, S, O, A

PART I

Part I has no answers.

PART II. History, Systems Review, Tests & Measures, Diagnosis, Prognosis

HISTORY: Demographics: Pt. is a 65 y.o. ♂ c̄ a dx of DJD
Ⓡ hip c̄ a THA on [date]. Physician is Dr. Sienn. Pt. is
Ⓡ - handed dominant. Current Condition: c/o Ⓡ hip pain
in area of sutures of the following intensities: 7 when moving, 3 when sitting, 2 when lying still (0 = no pain, 10 =
worst possible pain). Does not recall precautions for Pt.'s c̄
THA. PTA pain was constant & intensity was 9 or 10. Pt.
wants to eventually return to gardening & yard work

activities (Pt. goal). Social Hx: Lives c̄ his wife in his own
home. Plans to return home c̄ his wife p̄ D/C.
Employment/Work: Pt. is retired. Living Environment:
Has 1 step to enter home c̄ railing on Ⓡ ascending. Owns
a 3-in-1 commode, a walker, & a cane. General Health
Status: Pt. rates general health as good; no major life
changes in past yr. Social/Health Habits: Does not smoke;
only occasionally drinks ETOH. PTA attempted amb. for
exercise daily; was only able to amb. 1 block PTA. Two yrs.
Ago Pt. was able to amb. 1 mi. or more. Family Hx: Pt.'s
father died of MI @ age 78. Pt.'s mother died of breast CA
@ age 72. Pt. has no siblings. Medical/Surgical Hx: Hx of
htn. Hx of hospitalization for Ⓛ THA on 01/10/2000.
Functional Status/Activity Level: Immediately PTA, PT.
amb. s̄ assist. device. Hobby gardening. Gardens outside of
the church. Does volunteer ushering @ church.
Medications: Takes [antihypertensive medication].

SYSTEMS REVIEW: Cardiovascular/pulmonary: not
impaired. HR: 80 bpm. Resp. rate: 14 breaths/min. BP:
130/85. Edema: none noted. Integumentary: impaired.
Disruption: staples Ⓡ hip. Skin color: WNL. Skin texture:
not tested this date. Musculoskeletal: Gross symmetry not
impaired. Gross ROM & strength: impaired Ⓡ hip & knee.
Ht: 6 ft. 0 in. Wt: 185 lbs. Neuromuscular: Gait: impaired.
Locomotion: impaired transfers & bed mobility. Balance:
impaired in standing; uses walker. Not impaired in sitting.
Motor function: not impaired. Communication: not
impaired. Cognition: oriented × 3; not impaired. Learning
barriers: cannot read s̄ glasses. Education needs: home
exercise program, precautions for Pt.'s c̄ THA, progression
of recovery process, use of walker. ADLs including transfers. Learning style: prefers demonstration ā trying an
activity.

TESTS & MEASURES: Amb: Stood B/S c̄ walker 10%
PWB Ⓡ LE c̄ mod. assist. of 1. Transfers: Supine ↔ sit c̄
min. assist of 1. Sit ↔ stand & w/c ↔ mat pivot c̄ mod.
assist. of 1. Toilet transfers not tested this date. Ⓡ LE:
Strength grossly 1/5 in hip & knee musculature; ankle dorsiflexion 4+/5; ankle plantar flexion @ least 2/5 but not
tested further due to 10% PWB status. PROM: 0–20° hip
flexion, 0–10° hip abduction, 0° hip extension; adduction,
medical & lateral rotation of hip not tested due to hip precautions & recent surgery. Knee flexion: 0–70°. AROM:
Ⓡ ankle WNL. Incision Ⓡ hip 10 cm long over greater
trochanter; staples intact; healing well. UE & Ⓛ LE:
AROM WNL & strength 4+/5 throughout bilat. UEs &
Ⓛ LE. Group muscle testing performed UEs; individual
muscle testing performed LEs.

DIAGNOSIS: Indep. c̄ a walker is necessary for Pt. to
return to home. Impairments of ↓ ROM & strength Ⓡ LE
are preventing Pt. from indep. amb. on this date. Practice
Pattern: Musculoskeletal H: Impaired Joint Mobility,
Motor Function, Muscle Performance & ROM Associated c̄
Joint Arthroplasty.

PROGNOSIS: Pt. has good rehab. potential. His level to
function was good PTA & he has a great desire to return to
a healthy, active lifestyle in the community. Should be able
to return to home c̄ his wife indep. in amb. & a home exercise program to cont. to ↑ Ⓡ LE strength & ROM p̄ 3–4
days of therapy BID.

PART III. Problem, S, O, and A

Problem: Pt. is a 65 y.o. ♂ c̄ a dx of DJD Ⓡ hip c̄ a THA on [date]. Physician is Dr. Sienn. Hx of htn. Hx of hospitalization for Ⓛ THA on 01/10/2000. Takes [antihypertensive medication]. Pt. is Ⓡ handed dominant.

S: CURRENT CONDITION: c/o Ⓡ hip pain in area of sutures of the following intensities: 7 when moving, 3 when sitting, 2 when lying still (0 = no pain, 10 = worst possible pain). Does not recall precautions for Pt.'s c̄ THA. PTA pain was constant & intensity was 9 or 10. PT. GOALS: Pt. wants to eventually return to gardening & hard work activities (Pt. goal). SOCIAL HX: Lives c̄ his wife in his own home. Plans to return home c̄ his wife p̄ D/C. EMPLOYMENT/WORK: Pt. is retired. LIVING ENVIRONMENT: Has 1 step to enter home c̄ railing on Ⓡ ascending. Owns a 3-in-1 commode, a walker, & a cane. GENERAL HEALTH STATUS: Pt. rates general health as good; no major life changes in past yr. SOCIAL/HEALTH HABITS: Does not smoke; only occasionally drinks ETOH. PTA attempted amb. for exercise daily; was only able to amb. 1 block PTA. Two yrs. ago Pt. was able to amb. 1 mi. or more. FAMILY HX: Pt.'s father died of MI @ age 78. Pt.'s mother died of breast CA @ age 72. Pt. has no siblings. FUNCTIONAL STATUS/ACTIVITY LEVEL: Immediately PTA, PT. amb. s̄ assist. device. Hobby gardening. Gardens outside of the church. Does volunteer ushering @ church.

O: SYSTEMS REVIEW: Cardiovascular/pulmonary: not impaired. HR: 80 bpm. Resp. rate: 14 breaths/min. BP: 130/85. Edema: none noted. Integumentary: impaired. Disruption: staples Ⓡ hip. Skin color: WNL. Skin texture: not tested this date. Musculoskeletal: Gross symmetry not impaired. Gross ROM & strength: impaired Ⓡ hip & knee. Ht: 6 ft. 0 in. Wt: 185 lbs. Neuromuscular: Gait: impaired. Locomotion: impaired transfers & bed mobility. Balance: impaired in standing; uses walker. Not impaired in sitting. Motor function: not impaired. Communication: not impaired. Cognition: oriented × 3; not impaired. Learning barriers: cannot read s̄ glasses. Education needs: home exercise program, precautions for Pt.'s c̄ THA, progression of recovery process, use of walker, ADLs including transfers. Learning style: prefers demonstration ā trying an activity. AMB: Stood B/S c̄ walker 10% PWB Ⓡ LE c̄ mod. assist. of 1. TRANSFERS: Supine ↔ sit c̄ min. assist of 1. Sit ↔ stand & w/c ↔ mat pivot c̄ mod. assist. of 1. Toilet transfers not tested this date. Ⓡ LE: Strength grossly 1/5 in hip & knee musculature; ankle dorsiflexion 4+/5; ankle plantar flexion @ least 2/5 but not tested further due to 10% PWB status. PROM: 0–20° hip flexion, 0–10° hip abduction, 0° hip extension; adduction, medical & lateral rotation of hip not tested due to hip precautions & recent surgery. Knee flexion: 0–70°. AROM: Ⓡ ankle WNL. Incision Ⓡ hip 10 cm long over greater trochanter; staples intact; healing well. UE & Ⓛ LE: AROM WNL & strength 4+/5 throughout bilat. UEs & Ⓛ LE. Group muscle testing performed UEs; individual muscle testing performed LEs.

A: DIAGNOSIS: Indep. c̄ a walker is necessary for Pt. to return to home. Impairments of ↓ ROM & strength Ⓡ LE are preventing Pt. from indep. amb. on this date. Practice Pattern: Musculoskeletal H: Impaired Joint Mobility, Motor Function, Muscle Performance & ROM Associated c̄ Joint Arthroplasty.

PROGNOSIS: Pt. has good rehab. potential. His level to function was good PTA & he has a great desire to return to a healthy, active lifestyle in the community. Should be able to return to home c̄ his wife indep. in amb. & a home exercise program to cont. to ↑ Ⓡ LE strength & ROM p̄ 3–4 days of therapy BID.

Chapter 13:
Writing Expected Outcomes

● Worksheet 1

PART I

1. A. Pt. (implied)
    B. will manage & propel w/c
    C. a w/c must be present; Pt. must be @ home
    D. indep. (observable)
        ~ 50 ft. × 10 (measurable)
        within 1 mo. (time frame)
        (outcome is functional as it is written)
2. A. Pt.
    B. will demonstrate amb.
    C. c̄ prosthesis
        s̄ device
        stairs must be present
        uneven surfaces must be present
    D. on @ least 14 stairs (measurable)
        for @ least ¹/₂ mi. on even & uneven surfaces (measurable & observable)
        indep. (observable)
        within 2 wks. (time frame)
        to ensure Pt.'s ability to amb. in & out of his home & around his yard (functional)
3. A. Pt.
    B. will demonstrate body mechanics
    C. while lifting up to 50 lbs.
    D. body mechanics will be good (observable)
        To allow Pt. to return to work fully functional (function)
        within 4 wks. of Rx (time frame)
4. A. Pt.
    B. will demonstrate rolling
    C. Pt. must have a place to roll (implied)
    D. segmental rolling (observable)
        p̄ 6 mo. of Rx (time frame)
        to make Pt. more functional as she sleeps & plays (function)

PART II

1. Pt. will amb. c̄ crutches on level surfaces & 1 step elevation 40 ft. × 3 NWB Ⓛ LE indep. p̄ 2 days of Rx to allow Pt. to get around her house for ADL.
2. Pt. will demonstrate care & wrapping of her residual limb c̄ elastic wrap indep. applying even pressure 100% of the time to prepare for prosthetic training within 3 days.
3. Pt. will be able to lift a 5 lb. box from an overhead cupboard & place it on a table using bilat. UEs equally

within 2 mo. to enable Pt.'s ability to reach items on the shelves in her kitchen & closet @ home during ADL.

4. Pt. will amb. s̄ device in her home for 50 ft. × 4 using pursed lip breathing pattern within 4 wks. of Rx to enable her to cook & perform ADLs.

PART III

1. Pt. will be able to lift pots & pans up to 20 lbs. p̄ 10 visits to allow Pt. to lift pots & pans in her kitchen.
2. Pt. will be able to reach items in an overhead cabinet up to 5 ft. 10 in. p̄ 10 Rx sessions to allow Pt. to reach items in her overhead kitchen cabinets @ home.

Writing Expected Outcomes

● Worksheet 2

PART I

1. A. Pt. (implied)
   B. will amb.
   C. c̄ straight cane
       on level surfaces
       on @ least 5 stairs
   D. for 150 ft. × 2 (measurable)
       Indep. (observable)
       within 1 wk. (time span)
       so Pt.'s level of indep. @ home ↑ (function)
2. A. Pt.'s wife
   B. will transfer Pt. w/c ↔ supine in bed & w/c ↔ toilet
   C. w/c & bed must be present
   D. giving min. + 1 assist to Pt. (observable)
       indep. (observable)
       p̄ 1 mo. of Rx & 5 sessions of family teaching (time span)
       so wife can care for Pt. @ home (function)
3. A. Pt.
   B. will transfer w/c ↔ floor
   C. it is assumed w/c is present
   D. Indep. (observable)
       within 3 mo. (time frame)
       so Pt. can safely play on the floor c̄ her siblings (functional)

PART II

1. Pt. will sit on the edge of a mat or chair s̄ falling for @ least 10 min. p̄ 2 mo. of Rx to allow Pt. to more safely function @ school.
2. Pt. will transfer supine ↔ sit, sit ↔ stand, & on/off toilet c̄ raise toilet seat indep. p̄ 2 wks. of Rx for Pt. to function indep. @ home.
3. Pt. propel w/c on level surfaces, including tiled & carpeted surfaces indep. p̄ 1 mo. of Rx to ↑ Pt.'s indep. @ home.

PART III

1. Pt. will amb. c̄ a walker FWB as tolerated on level surfaces & 3 stairs c̄ a handrail in 2 wks. to allow Pt. to be safe in amb. as he returns home.

2. Pt. will transfer bed ↔ chair, sit ↔ stand & on/off commode indep. p̄ 2 wks. of Rx to allow Pt. to function @ home alone.

C h a p t e r   1 4 :
Writing Anticipated Goals

● Worksheet 1

PART I

1. A. Pt. (implied)
   B. will ↑ Ⓡ shoulder flexion AROM
   C. (assumed you will measure AROM with a goniometer)
   D. to 0–90° (measurable)
       within 6 Rx sessions (time frame)
       to work toward Pt. reaching her overhead kitchen cupboards (function)
2. A. Pt.
   B. will grasp object
   C. object will be in midline
   D. 3 out of 4 times (measurable)
       within 3 mo. (time span)
       to ↑ Pt.'s functional use of UEs during ADLs (function)
3. A. Pt.
   B. will demonstrate good body mechanics
   C. by performance of tasks in obstacle course
   D. correct performance of @ least 90% of tasks (measurable & observable)
       p̄ 3 Rx sessions (time span)
       to prevent further Pt. injury @ work (function)

PART II

1. Pt. will amb. c̄ a walker NWB Ⓛ LE ~100 ft. × 2 indep. on level surfaces only p̄ 1 wk. of Rx.
2. Pt.'s wife & son will transfer Pt. w/c ↔ supine in bed indep. p̄ 4 family training sessions to care for Pt. @ home.
3. Pt. will wrap residual limb c̄ 3 in. elastic wrap c̄ verbal cues for placement of elastic wrap p̄ 5 Rx sessions to prepare for prosthetic training.

PART III

1. (Case 1) Pt. will don and doff prosthesis c̄ SBA of 1 person p̄ 1 wk. of Rx to assist c̄ sit ↔ stand transfers.
2. (Case 2) Pt. will be able to stand in // bars c̄ @ least 50% of body wt. shifted onto Ⓛ LE c̄ min. assist. of 1 & verbal cues p̄ 1 wk. of Rx.
3. (Case 3) Pt. will be pain free in prone on elbows position for 5 min. p̄ 2 Rx to work on performance of ADLs.

PART IV

1. Degree (time span, measurable factors)
2. Degree (time span, measurable or observable factor—could be assumed to be 100% of the time correctly, some tie to function is needed)
3. Audience, behavior (who will do what?)

Writing Anticipated Goals

● Worksheet 2

PART I

1. A. Pt.
   B. will ↑ cardiopulmonary endurance
   C. p̄ amb. s̄ device for 150 ft.
   D. as demonstrated by max. ↑ of resp. rate of 5 breaths/min. (measurable)
      p̄ 6 Rx sessions (time span)
      to (Pt. function @ home (function)
2. A. Pt.
   B. will be able to long sit
   C. propped c̄ a pillow or wedge
   D. maintaining good head position 0–45° of neck flexion (measurable/observable)
      for 1 min. (measurable)
      within 6 wks. of Rx (time span)
      to assist. c̄ Pt. function in the classroom (function)
3. A. Pt.
   B. will transfer supine ↔ sit on a mat
   C. mat must be there
   D. using rotation & pushing c̄ his UEs (1 out of 3 attempts correct) (observable & measurable)
      within 1 mo. (time span)

PART II

1. Pt. will hold his head in midline while in supine for 15 sec. within 3 mo. of Rx.
2. Pt. will roll supine ↔ prone on a mat indep. in 6–8 wks.
3. Pt. will amb. 50% PWB (R) LE on 5 stairs c̄ a walker c̄ min. assist. from his wife p̄ 1 wk. of Rx.

PART III

1. (Case 1)
   1. Pt. will perform 7 reps of both UE PNF patterns within available AROM p̄ 1 wk. of Rx.
   2. ↑ (R) shoulder flexion AROM to 100° p̄ 1 wk. of Rx.
   3. ↑ (L) shoulder flexion AROM to 90° p̄ 1 wk. of Rx.
   4. ↑ strength throughout bilat. UEs to 3+/5 within available AROM p̄ 1 wk. of Rx.
   5. Pt. will be able to retrieve items .5 lbs. in wt. from the lower shelf of overhead cabinet p̄ 1 wk. of Rx.
2. (Case 2) ↑ cervical rotation to 10° bilat. in 2 days.
3. (Case 3) Pt. will amb. NWB (R) LE for 40 ft. × 2 on level surfaces c̄ min. assist. of 1 person in 1 wk.

PART IV

1. Degree (time span), Audience (could be assumed)
2. Degree (how much AROM is expected? Also, tying it to function would be helpful), Audience (could be assumed)
3. Audience, Behavior (ambulate?), Condition (wt. bearing status?), Degree (time span, # of stairs)

C h a p t e r 1 5 : Writing the Intervention Plan

● Worksheet 1

PART I

1. IP
2. AG
3. IP
4. IP
5. AG
6. IP
7. AG
8. IP
9. AG
10. EO

PART II

1. Pt. will be seen OD for hot pack for 20 min. to lumbar area.
2. Pt. will be seen 3×/wk. for continuous US @ 1.0 W/cm² for 7 min. to (R) upper trapezius
3. Pt. will be seen BID to progress Pt. through knee exercise program for bilat. knees (attached).

PART III

1. How often
   For how long
   Setting of the pump
   To what (UE? LE? Which one?)
2. For how long
   Which whirlpool?
   Temperature?
   Whirlpool additive
   To which part of the body
   Some facilities list type of agitation (full, mild, direct, or indirect)

Writing the Intervention Plan

● Worksheet 2

PART I

1. IP
2. EO
3. IP
4. EO
5. IP
6. AG
7. AG
8. AG
9. AG
10. IP
11. IP

PART II

1. 3×/wk as an OP: Pulsed US to (R) shoulder @ 1.5 W/cm² for 7 min. Mobilization to (R) shoulder. Ice pack for 20 min. @ end of Rx session. Pt. will be instructed

in & given a copy of home exercise program (attached). Will seek OT referral for ADL evaluation. [Rationale for referral to OT should be in the Diagnosis portion of the note.]

2. BID: Gait training c̄ axillary crutches NWB Ⓡ LE. Transfer training sit ↔ stand, supine ↔ sit & on/off toilet. AROM exercise to LEs beginning c̄ 10 reps ea. exercise & ↑ to 30 reps × 3 sets. Pt. will be instructed in proper care of residual limb. Pt. will be instructed in wrapping his residual limb.

Final Review Worksheet Answers
Patient/Client Management Note: Examination, Evaluation & Plan of Care
SOAP Note: Problem, S, O, A, & P

PART II

11/08/2002: HISTORY: <u>Demographics:</u> Pt. is a 16 y.o. ♀ Pt. of Dr. Gungo. Medical dx: fx Ⓡ distal tibia & fx Ⓡ prox. humerus. ORIF Ⓡ proximal humerus on (date). Cast applied to Ⓡ leg & sling applied Ⓡ UE. Pt. is Ⓡ-hand dominant. <u>Current Condition:</u> c/o pain Ⓡ ankle of an intensity of 10/10 when Ⓡ LE was initially in a dependent position (0 = no pain, 10 = worst possible pain). Pain Ⓡ ankle subsided p̄ Pt. put Ⓡ LE in a dependent position multiple times. Also c/o pain of 7/10 in Ⓡ shoulder c̄ Ⓡ elbow AAROM. Pt. reports difficulty feeding herself & cannot dress herself; states has not seen OT. Pt. was in a car accident c̄ 1 friend; the friend was driving & is currently in the community s̄ injury @ this time. Pt. wants to return to school ASAP p̄ D/C. <u>Social hx:</u> Lives c̄ both parents. Parents both work so Pt. will be @ home alone @ D/C until she can go to school. Parents state insurance will rent a w/c for Pt. use until she is healed. <u>Employment status:</u> Pt. is a high school student. School is very academically challenging & competitive & Pt. does not believe she can stay out of school until she is healed. School is on 1 level c̄ no steps to enter. Distances between classrooms < or = 1500 ft. Has 7 class periods/day. Floor surfaces are linoleum throughout the school. <u>Living environment:</u> Lives in a 1-story house c̄ 1 step @ entrance s̄ handrail. Home has carpeted floor surfaces throughout. <u>General health status:</u> Pt. & parents report Pt. on swim team @ school; swims daily all year & general health is good. <u>Social/health habits:</u> Pt. does not smoke or drink ETOH. <u>Family health hx:</u> Htn. both parents controlled by medication. <u>Pt.'s medical/surgical hx:</u> No previous hospitalizations or serious illnesses. <u>Medications:</u> Pt. is currently taking [pain medication]; takes no other medications regularly. <u>Other clinical tests:</u> X-ray: good alignment of Ⓡ LE fx in cast & of Ⓡ humerus p̄ surgery.

SYSTEMS REVIEW: <u>Cardiopulmonary:</u> not impaired. BP: 110/70; HR: 70 bpm; Resp. rate: 12/breaths min. No edema noted. <u>Integumentary:</u> impaired. Disruption of skin @ incision site Ⓡ upper arm. Continuity of skin color: bruising noted Ⓡ UE & Ⓡ foot. Pliability: not impaired Ⓛ extremities; Ⓡ extremities not tested this date. <u>Musculoskeletal:</u> impaired. Gross symmetry not impaired sitting; cannot stand. Gross ROM: impaired Ⓡ UE & LE.

Gross strength: impaired Ⓡ UE & LE. Height: 5' 6", weight 125 lbs. <u>Neuromuscular:</u> Gait: impaired. Locomotion: impaired. Balance: not impaired sitting; cannot stand. Motor function: not impaired. <u>Communication:</u> not impaired; age appropriate. <u>Cognition:</u> not impaired; oriented × 3. <u>Learning barriers:</u> none. <u>Learning style:</u> Pt. best learns by listening as she tries an activity. <u>Education needs:</u> healing process of incision; adaptation of home to w/c; w/c management; w/c propulsion; ADLs; safety c̄ w/c; home exercise program for Ⓡ UE.

TESTS & MEASURES: <u>Transfers:</u> sit ↔ stand & w/c ↔ bed c̄ max. assist of 1 NWB Ⓡ LE & UE. Supine ↔ sit c̄ mod. assist. of 1 person. Toilet transfers not tested this date. <u>W/c Management:</u> Unable to manage Ⓡ w/c brakes or leg rest. <u>W/c propulsion:</u> propelled w/c 10 ft. using Ⓛ LE & UE c̄ min. assist. of 1 person & verbal cues. Was too exhausted to continue further. Ⓛ LE & UE: WNL AROM & strength throughout. Ⓡ UE: Bruising noted throughout entire Ⓡ UE. Ⓡ shoulder not examined due to recent fx. Ⓡ elbow AAROM: 30–70°. Ⓡ hand & wrist AROM WNL when Pt. is given verbal cues to complete full ROM; performed very slowly. Strength Ⓡ biceps and triceps: 2/5. Strength of musculature controlling Ⓡ wrist & hand is 3/5. Ⓡ LE: Bruising noted Ⓡ toes. Toes warm & color WNL. AROM WNL @ hip & knee. Strength 5/5 Ⓡ hip & knee musculature. Able to wiggle toes. Short leg cast Ⓡ ankle & foot so not examined this date.

DIAGNOSIS: Rigorous AROM Ⓡ elbow, wrist, & hand are needed to prevent loss of all strength & ROM. Pt.'s lack of mobility is due to inability to use Ⓡ extremities due to recent fx. A referral to OT is essential to Pt.'s rehab. process to assist. her c̄ eating, bathing, dressing, & managing items for return to school in a w/c. <u>Practice Pattern:</u> Musculoskeletal G: Impaired Joint Mobility, Muscle Performance & ROM Associated c̄ Fx.

PROGNOSIS: Pt. has excellent rehab. potential. Will be able to return home & to school c̄ 2 wks. of rehab. Pt. cannot stay @ home alone until she becomes indep. in w/c propulsion & transfers. Pt. will need assist. in propelling her w/c over 500 ft. @ school.

EXPECTED OUTCOMES: to be achieved p̄ 2 wks. of PT
1. Pt. will indep. transfer supine ↔ sit, sit ↔ stand, w/c ↔ bed NWB Ⓡ LE & UE to be functional @ home & school.
2. Pt. will indep. manage w/c brakes & footrests to function @ home & school.
3. Pt. will propel w/c for 500 ft. × 2 indep. using Ⓛ UE & LE to function @ school.
4. Pt. will prevent loss of function in Ⓡ elbow, wrist, & fingers to maximize UE function p̄ Ⓡ humerus is healed.

ANTICIPATED GOALS: To be achieved p̄ 1 wk. of PT
1. Pt. will transfer supine ↔ sit c̄ verbad cues.
2. Pt. will transfer sit ↔ stand c̄ min. assist. of 1.
3. Pt. will transfer w/c ↔ bed & on/off toilet c̄ mod. assist. of 1 person.
4. Pt. will manage w/c brakes & footrest using an extended Ⓡ brake lever c̄ verbal cues.
5. Pt. will propel w/c for ~100 ft. using Ⓛ UE & LE.
6. Pt. will be indep. in performing home exercise program for AROM of Ⓡ elbow, wrist & fingers.

INTERVENTION PLAN: Will see Pt. BID @ B/S. Will train Pt. in transfers supine ↔ sit, sit ↔ stand, w/c ↔ bed & on/off toilet. Will train Pt. in w/c management & propulsion. Will teach Pt. a home exercise program for AROM to Ⓡ elbow, wrist, & fingers & will give Pt. a copy of program (attached); Pt. will perform the exercise program 3×/day, 1× c̄ PT supervision & 2× indep. – (your name), SPT

PART III

Problem: Pt. is a 16 y.o. ♀ Pt. of Dr. Gungo. Pt. is Ⓡ-hand dominant. Medical dx: fx Ⓡ distal tibia & fx Ⓡ prox. humerus. ORIF Ⓡ proximal humerus on (date). Cast applied to Ⓡ leg & sling applied Ⓡ UE. Other clinical tests: X-ray: good alignment of Ⓡ LE fx in cast & of Ⓡ humerus p̄ surgery. Medications: Pt. is currently taking [pain medication]; takes no other medications regularly.

S: Current Condition: c/o pain Ⓡ ankle of an intensity of 10/10 when Ⓡ LE was initially in a dependent position (0 = no pain, 10 = worst possible pain). Pain Ⓡ ankle subsided p̄ Pt. put Ⓡ LE in a dependent position multiple times. Also c/o pain of 7/10 in Ⓡ shoulder c̄ Ⓡ elbow AAROM. Pt. reports difficulty feeding herself & cannot dress herself; states has not seen OT. Pt. was in a car accident c̄ 1 friend; the friend was driving & is currently in the community s̄ injury @ this time. Pt. goals: Pt. wants to return to school ASAP p̄ D/C. Social hx: Lives c̄ both parents. Parents both work so Pt. will be @ home alone @ D/C until she can go to school. Parents state insurance will rent a w/c for Pt. use until she is healed. Employment status: Pt. is a high school student. School is very academically challenging & competitive & Pt. does not believe she can stay out of school until she is healed. School is on 1 level c̄ no steps to enter. Distances between classrooms ≤ 1500 ft. Has 7 class periods/day. Floor surfaces are linoleum throughout the school. Living environment: Lives in a 1-story house c̄ 1 step @ entrance s̄ handrail. Home has carpeted floor surfaces throughout. General health status: Pt. & parents report Pt. on swim team @ school; swims daily all year & general health is good. Social/health habits: Pt. does not smoke or drink ETOH. Family health hx: Htn. both parents controlled by medication. Pt.'s medical/surgical hx: No previous hospitalizations or serious illnesses.

O: SYSTEMS REVIEW: Cardiopulmonary: not impaired. BP: 110/70; HR: 70 bpm; Resp. rate: 12/breaths min. No edema noted. Integumentary: impaired. Disruption of skin @ incision site Ⓡ upper arm. Continuity of skin color: bruising noted Ⓡ UE & Ⓡ foot. Pliability: not impaired Ⓛ extremities; Ⓡ extremities not tested this date. Musculoskeletal: impaired. Gross symmetry not impaired sitting; cannot stand. Gross ROM: impaired Ⓡ UE & LE. Gross strength: impaired Ⓡ UE & LE. Height: 5′6″, weight 125 lbs. Neuromuscular: Gait: impaired. Locomotion: impaired. Balance: not impaired sitting; cannot stand. Motor function: not impaired. Communication: not impaired; age appropriate. Cognition: not impaired; oriented × 3. Learning barriers: none. Learning style: Pt. best learns by listening as she tries an activity. Education needs: healing process of incision; adaptation of home to w/c; w/c manage-

ment; w/c propulsion; ADLs; safety c̄ w/c; home exercise program for Ⓡ UE. TRANSFERS: sit ↔ stand & w/c ↔ bed c̄ max. assist of 1 NWB Ⓡ LE & UE. Supine ↔ sit c̄ mod. assist. of 1 person. Toilet transfers not tested this date. W/C MANAGEMENT: Unable to manage Ⓡ w/c brakes or leg rest. W/C PROPULSION: propelled w/c 10 ft. using Ⓛ LE & UE c̄ min. assist. of 1 person & verbal cues. Was too exhausted to continue further. Ⓛ LE & UE: WNL AROM & strength throughout. Ⓡ UE: Bruising noted throughout entire Ⓡ UE. Ⓡ shoulder not examined due to recent fx. Ⓡ elbow AAROM: 30–70°. Ⓡ hand & wrist AROM WNL when Pt. is given verbal cues to complete full ROM; performed very slowly. Strength Ⓡ biceps and triceps: 2/5. Strength of musculature controlling Ⓡ wrist & hand is 3/5. Ⓡ LE: Bruising noted Ⓡ toes. Toes warm & color WNL. AROM WNL @ hip & knee. Strength 5/5 Ⓡ hip & knee musculature. Able to wiggle toes. Short leg cast Ⓡ ankle & foot, so not examined this date.

A: DIAGNOSIS: Rigorous AROM Ⓡ elbow, wrist, & hand are needed to prevent loss of all strength & ROM. Pt.'s lack of mobility is due to inability to use Ⓡ extremities due to recent fx. A referral to OT is essential to Pt.'s rehab. process to assist. her c̄ eating, bathing, dressing, & managing items for return to school in a w/c. Practice Pattern: Musculoskeletal G: Impaired Joint Mobility, Muscle Performance & ROM Associated c̄ Fx. PROGNOSIS: Pt. has excellent rehab. potential. Will be able to return home & to school c̄ 2 wks. of rehab. Pt. cannot stay @ home alone until she becomes indep. in w/c propulsion & transfers. Pt. will need assist. in propelling her w/c over 500 ft. @ school.

Plan of Care: EXPECTED OUTCOMES: to be achieved p̄ 2 wks. of PT

1. Pt. will indep. transfer supine ↔ sit, sit ↔ stand, w/c ↔ bed NWB Ⓡ LE & UE to be functional @ home & school.
2. Pt. will indep. manage w/c brakes & footrests to function @ home & school.
3. Pt. will propel w/c for 500 ft. × 2 indep. using Ⓛ UE & LE to function @ school.
4. Pt. will prevent loss of function in Ⓡ elbow, wrist, & fingers to maximize UE function p̄ Ⓡ humerus is healed.

ANTICIPATED GOALS: To be achieved p̄ 1 wk. of PT
1. Pt. will transfer supine ↔ sit c̄ verbal cues.
2. Pt. will transfer sit ↔ stand c̄ min. assist. of 1.
3. Pt. will transfer w/c ↔ bed & on/off toilet c̄ mod. assist. of 1 person.
4. Pt. will manage w/c brakes & footrest using an extended Ⓡ brake lever c̄ verbal cues.
5. Pt. will propel w/c for ~100 ft. using Ⓛ UE & LE.
6. Pt. will be indep. in performing home exercise program for AROM of Ⓡ elbow, wrist, & fingers.

INTERVENTION PLAN: Will see Pt. BID @ B/S. Will train Pt. in transfers supine ↔ sit, sit ↔ stand, w/c ↔ bed & on/off toilet. Will train Pt. in w/c management & propulsion. Will teach Pt. a home exercise program for AROM to Ⓡ elbow, wrist, & fingers & will give Pt. a copy of program (attached); Pt. will perform the exercise program 3×/day, 1× c̄ PT supervision & 2× indep. – (your name), SPT

Note Writing and the Process of Clinical Decision-Making

Patient/Client Management Note	Patient/Client Management Process	SOAP Note
	EXAMINATION	
History Systems Review Tests & Measures	↓	Problem Subjective Objective (includes Systems Review subsection)
	EVALUATION	A (Assessment) (includes the following subsections:)
Diagnosis Prognosis	↓	Diagnosis Prognosis
	PLAN OF CARE	Plan of Care (includes the following subsections:
Expected Outcomes		Expected Outcomes (in some facilities, included under A)
Anticipated Goals		Anticipated Goals (in some facilities, included under A)
Interventions, including Patient Education	↓	Interventions, including Patient Education
	OUTCOMES (re-examination occurs & another note is written at the time of re-examination)	

Summary of the Patient/Client Management Note Contents

▌Initial Note

History

- **Identifying information** (patient's name, address, admission date, date of birth, sex, dominant hand, race, ethnicity, language, education level, advance directive preferences, referral source, and reasons for referral to therapy)

- **Current conditions/chief complaints** (onset date of the problem, any incident that caused or contributed to the onset of the problem, prior history of similar problems, how the patient is caring for the problem, what makes the problem better and worse, patient goals for therapy, and any other practitioner the patient is seeing for the problem)

- **Social history** (cultural/religious beliefs that might affect care, the person(s) with whom the patient lived prior to admission and will live with at discharge, available social and physical supports the patient has now and will have at discharge, and the availability of a caregiver)

- **Employment status** (full time or part time, inside or outside of the home, retired or a student, description of the workplace and/or workplace demands)

- **Living environment** (devices and equipment the patient uses, the type of residence, information about the environment such as stairs or ramps available, and past use of community services such as day services or program, home-health services, homemaking services, hospice, Meals on Wheels, mental health services, respiratory therapy, or one of the rehabilitation therapies)

- **General health status** (patient's rating of his or her health and whether the patient has experienced any major life changes during the past year)

- **Social/health habits** (past and current alcohol and tobacco use and exercise habits)

- **Family health history** (family history of heart disease, hypertension, stroke, diabetes, cancer, psychological conditions, arthritis, osteoporosis, and other conditions)

- **Patient's medical/surgical history**

- **Functional status/activity level** (everything from bed mobility, transfers, gait, self-care, home management, and community and work activities that apply to the patient's current situation or condition)

- **Medications** the patient takes

- **Growth and development** (developmental history of a patient)

- **Other clinical tests** (laboratory or radiologic tests, the dates of those tests, and the findings of those tests)

Systems Review

- **Cardiovascular/Pulmonary** (heart rate, respiratory rate, blood pressure, or edema): listed as impaired or not impaired; individual measurements of heart rate, blood pressure, respiratory rate and a general description of edema are listed

- **Integumentary System** (integumentary disruption, continuity of skin color, skin pliability or texture): listed as impaired or not impaired

- **Musculoskeletal System:** gross symmetry during standing, sitting, and activities; gross range of motion; gross muscle strength; each listed as impaired or unimpaired; height and weight are recorded

- **Neuromuscular System:** gait, locomotion (transfers, bed mobility), balance, and motor function (motor control, motor learning) are each listed as impaired or unimpaired

- **Communication Style or Abilities** (including age-appropriate communication): listed as impaired or unimpaired

- **Affect** (emotional/behavioral responses): listed as impaired or unimpaired
- **Cognition** (whether the patient is oriented to person, place and time [oriented × 3] or the patient's level of consciousness): listed as impaired or unimpaired
- **Learning Barriers:** notes difficulty with vision, hearing, inability to read, inability to understand what is read, language barriers (needs an interpreter) and any other learning barrier noted by the therapist
- **Learning Style:** notes how the patient/client best learns (pictures, reading, listening, demonstration, other)
- **Education Needs:** reports areas in which the patient needs more education or information (disease process, safety, use of devices/equipment, activities of daily living, exercise program, recovery and healing process, and other education needs)

Tests and Measures

Items in the Tests and Measures section should have the following attributes:

- Be a result of tests and measures performed by the therapist or an observation made by the therapist
- Be listed in a subcategory that organizes the information in a logical manner, either by test performed or functional activity observed, or by part of the body reported

Diagnosis

The Diagnosis section may include any of the following:

- A description of the relationship between examination findings, including inconsistencies between examination findings
- A description of how impairments relate to the functional deficits
- A description of how functional deficits keep the patient from functioning in his or her specific environment
- A brief summary of the examination findings that led the therapist to place the patient in a specific practice pattern or movement dysfunction diagnosis
- A listing of testing procedures that would be helpful but could not be completed during the initial therapy session
- A listing of reasons for referral to another practitioner
- Placement of patient's deficits in primary and at times secondary practice patterns/movement dysfunction diagnostic categories

Prognosis

The Prognosis section may include any of the following:

- The patient's rehabilitation potential
- A prediction of a level of improvement in function and the amount of time needed to reach the level
- A discussion of factors influencing the prognosis such as living environment, patient's condition prior to the onset of the current therapy diagnosis, and current illnesses or medical conditions
- A justification of unusual expected outcomes or anticipated goals
- A justification for further therapy for a patient who appears relatively independent with one functional activity
- A discussion of the patient's progress in therapy (why the patient failed to progress as quickly as predicted, why a patient suddenly regressed, or why a patient suddenly progressed more quickly than predicted)
- A discussion or listing of future services needed

Expected Outcomes

1. State the long term expected outcomes of therapy.
2. Outcomes are generally functional.
3. Outcomes are based on discussion during the Diagnosis and Prognosis parts of the note.
4. Outcomes are the basis for setting Anticipated Goals.

Components of Expected Outcomes

1. **Audience:** The patient, a family member, or the patient with a family member (sometimes implied)

2. **Behavior:** An action verb, often followed by the object of the behavior
3. **Condition:** The circumstances under which the behavior must be done or the conditions necessary for the behavior to occur (sometimes implied)
4. **Degree:** The minimal number, the percentage or proportion, limitation or departure from a fixed standard, or distinguishing features of successful performance; always includes a time span for achievement of the outcome and a tie to the patient's function in his environment

Anticipated Goals

1. Goals are the steps along the way to achieving expected outcomes.
2. Goals are based on the expected outcomes.
3. Goals serve as the basis for setting the Intervention Plan.

The components of anticipated goals are the same as those of expected outcomes. Anticipated goals differ from expected outcomes in the following ways:

1. The time span is not as long.
2. Anticipated goals are not as frequently expressed in functional terms in some facilities.
3. Anticipated goals are frequently revised.

Intervention Plan

The Intervention Plan must include the following information:

1. Frequency per day or per week that the patient will be seen (or the total number of visits that the therapist will see the patient).
2. The intervention the patient will receive.

Also frequently included are the following:

1. The location of the intervention
2. The intervention progression
3. Plans for further examination or re-examination
4. Plans for discharge
5. Plans for patient and/or family education
6. Equipment needs and equipment ordered for or sold to the patient

▌Interim/Progress Notes

History

Includes updates or additional information regarding the patient's status since the most recent note was written.

Systems Review

Usually not included unless the patient's condition changes.

Tests and Measures

Tests and measures are updated or added to the information reported in the initial note or last interim note.

Diagnosis

Usually discussed in an Interim Note, or Progress Note, only if the therapy diagnosis has changed, referral to another practitioner has been made or recommended, or if the patient's functional activities or impairments change to fit a different primary or secondary practice pattern or movement dysfunction category.

Prognosis

Prognosis is usually only mentioned if the prognosis changes because of a change in the patient's condition.

Expected Outcomes

Expected Outcomes usually are not addressed in interim notes unless they have been achieved or need to be revised.

Anticipated Goals

Interim notes refer to the anticipated goals achieved and set new anticipated goals. If a goal has not yet been achieved, the notes comment on the reason the anticipated goal has not been achieved and reset the goal to make it more reasonable or restate the same goal to include a new time span.

Intervention Plan

The intervention plan needs to be revised as the patient's condition is re-examined and new anticipated goals are set.

▍Discharge Notes

History

Includes updates or additional information regarding the patient's status since the most recent note was written *or* completely summarizes the history of the patient from the initial note through discharge, whether the patient feels the goals set were achieved, and whether the patient feels ready to function at home or work.

Systems Review

In the Discharge Notes, the Systems Review is either not mentioned at all *or* completely summarizes the Systems Review written in the initial note.

Tests and Measures

The Discharge Summary updates the patient's status since the last note was written *or* completely summarizes the patient's condition upon discharge from the facility (more similar to the initial note in format and length).

Diagnosis

Diagnosis may include the following:

1. A discussion of the progression of the patient through diagnostic categories and/or movement dysfunction diagnoses *or* a diagnosis section similar to the initial note
2. Referrals made to other health professionals

Prognosis

Prognosis may include the following:

1. A discussion of suggested further therapy
2. A discussion of whether or not the patient achieved the expected outcomes and whether anticipated goals may occur

Expected Outcomes

The discharge summary indicates which of the expected outcomes have been achieved and which have not been achieved (and why they were not achieved).

Anticipated Goals

In some facilities, comments are made on the most recently set anticipated goals and why they were or were not achieved. In other facilities, no comment is made on the anticipated goals.

Intervention Plan

The following information should be briefly stated:

1. Interventions delivered
2. If instruction in a home program was done and the patient's/caregiver's level of independence in the program
3. If any other type of instruction of the patient or family was performed and the level of learning that occurred (in observable terms)
4. If the patient was sold any type of equipment
5. If written instructions for any equipment sold to the patient were given
6. The number of times the patient was seen in therapy
7. Any instances of the patient skipping or canceling treatment sessions
8. If and when the patient was not seen or was put on hold, and why
9. To where the patient was discharged
10. The reason from discharge from PT
11. Recommendations for follow-up interventions or care given to the patient

Summary of the SOAP Note Contents

▌Problem

The Problem part of the note contains the following:

- **Medical diagnosis/present conditions/diseases** affecting the present condition/treatment
- **Demographic information** (patient's name, address, admission date, date of birth, sex, dominant hand, race, ethnicity, language, education level, advance directive preferences, referral source, and reasons for referral to therapy)
- **Recent or past surgeries** affecting the present condition/treatment
- **Past conditions/diseases** affecting the present condition/treatment
- **Medical test results** affecting the present condition/treatment

▌Subjective (S)

The Subjective part of the note contains information that the patient and/or significant others tell the therapist or assistant such as:

- **Current conditions/chief complaints** (the onset date of the problem, any incident that caused or contributed to the onset of the problem, prior history of similar problems, how the patient is caring for the problem, what makes the problem better and worse, and any other practitioner the patient is seeing for the problem)
- **Functional status/activity level** (activities that the patient can no longer perform as a result of the patient's current condition; includes bed mobility, transfers, gait, self-care, home management, and community and work activities that apply to the patient's current situation or condition)

- **Social history** (cultural/religious beliefs that might affect care, the person(s) with whom the patient lived prior to admission and will live with at discharge, available social and physical supports the patient has now and will have at discharge, and the availability of a caregiver)
- **Employment status** (full time or part time, inside or outside of the home, retired or student, work place demands and set up)
- **Living environment** (devices and equipment the patient uses, the type of residence in which the patient lives, information about the living environment such as stairs or ramps available, past use of community services including day services or programs, home-health services, homemaking services, hospice, Meals on Wheels, mental health services, respiratory therapy, or one of the rehabilitation therapies)
- **General health status** (rating of the patient's health and whether the patient has experienced any major life changes during the past year)
- **Social/health habits** (past and current alcohol and tobacco use and exercise habits)
- **Family health history** (heart disease, hypertension, stroke, diabetes, cancer, psychological conditions, arthritis, osteoporosis, and other conditions)
- **Patient's medical/surgical history**
- **Medications** that the patient currently takes
- **Growth and development** (developmental history of a patient; most applicable to pediatric patients)
- **Other clinical tests** (laboratory or radiologic tests, the dates of those tests, and the findings of those tests)
- **Response to treatment interventions**
- **Patient goals** for therapy

▌Objective (O)

The Objective part of the note must include the following:

Systems Review

- **Cardiovascular/Pulmonary** (heart rate, respiratory rate, blood pressure or edema): listed as impaired or not impaired; individual measurements of heart rate, blood pressure, respiratory rate, and a general description of edema are listed

- **Integumentary System** (integumentary disruption, continuity of skin color, skin pliability or texture): listed as impaired or not impaired

- **Musculoskeletal System:** gross symmetry during standing, sitting, and activities; gross range of motion; gross muscle strength; each listed as impaired or unimpaired; height and weight are recorded

- **Neuromuscular System:** gait, locomotion (transfers, bed mobility), balance, and motor function (motor control, motor learning); each are listed as impaired or unimpaired

- **Communication Style or Abilities** (including age-appropriate communication): listed as impaired or unimpaired

- **Affect** (emotional and behavioral responses): listed as impaired or unimpaired

- **Cognition** (whether the patient is oriented to person, place and time [oriented × 3] or the patient's level of consciousness): listed as impaired or unimpaired

- **Learning Barriers:** notes difficulty with vision, hearing, inability to read, inability to understand what is read, language barriers (needs an interpreter), and any other learning barrier noted by the therapist

- **Learning Style:** notes how the patient/client best learns (pictures, reading, listening, demonstration, other)

- **Education Needs:** reports areas in which the patient needs more education or information (disease process, safety, use of devices/equipment, activities of daily living, exercise program, recovery/healing process and other education needs)

The Objective part of the note also includes any of the following information (depending on the individual clinical facility):

1. Information that is a result of tests and measures (must be measurable and reproducible data; may use database, flow sheets, or charts, and summarize data under Objective)
2. Part of the interventions already given to a patient (particularly specific exercises taught to the patient, the level of independence in performing the exercises, number of repetitions tolerated, positions used, modifications necessary)
3. Functional information; this information is usually stated first in the Objective part of the note.

Items in the Objective section should meet the following criteria:

- Be a result of tests and measures performed by the therapist or an observation made by the therapist

- Be listed in a subcategory that organizes the information in a logical manner, either by test performed/functional activity observed or by part of the body reported

▌Assessment (A)

The Assessment part of the note has two subsections: Diagnosis and Prognosis.

Diagnosis

The Diagnosis section may include any of the following:

- A description of the relationship between examination findings, including inconsistencies between examination findings

- A description of how impairments relate to the functional deficits

- A description of how functional deficits keep the patient from functioning in his specific environment

- A brief summary of the examination findings that led the therapist to place the patient in a specific practice pattern or movement dysfunction diagnosis

- A listing of testing procedures that would be helpful but could not be completed during the initial therapy session

- A listing of reasons for referral to another practitioner
- Placement of patient's deficits in primary and at times secondary practice patterns/movement dysfunction diagnostic categories

Prognosis

The Prognosis section may include any of the following:

- The patient's rehabilitation potential
- A prediction of a level of improvement in function and the amount of time needed to reach that level
- A discussion of factors influencing the prognosis such as living environment, patient's condition prior to the onset of the current therapy diagnosis, and current illnesses or medical conditions
- A justification of unusual expected outcomes or anticipated goals
- A justification for further therapy for a patient who appears relatively independent with one functional activity
- A discussion of the patient's progress in therapy (why the patient failed to progress as quickly as predicted, why a patient suddenly regressed, or why a patient suddenly progressed more quickly than predicted)
- A discussion or listing of future services needed

▌Plan of Care (P)

The Plan of Care part of the note has three subsections: Expected Outcomes, Anticipated Goals, and Interventions or Intervention Plan.

Expected Outcomes

1. State the long term expected outcomes of therapy.
2. Outcomes are generally functional.
3. Outcomes are based on discussion during the Diagnosis and Prognosis parts of the note.
4. Outcomes are the basis for setting Anticipated Goals.

Components of Expected Outcomes

1. **Audience:** The patient, a family member, or the patient with a family member (sometimes implied)

2. **Behavior:** An action verb, often followed by the object of the behavior
3. **Condition:** The circumstances under which the behavior must be done or the conditions necessary for the behavior to occur (sometimes implied).
4. **Degree:** The minimal number, the percentage or proportion, limitation or departure from a fixed standard, or distinguishing features of successful performance; always includes a time span for achievement of the outcome and a tie to the patient's function in his environment.

Anticipated Goals

1. Goals are the steps along the way to achieving expected outcomes.
2. Goals are based on the expected outcomes.
3. Goals serve as the basis for setting the Intervention Plan.

The components of anticipated goals are the same as those of expected outcomes. Anticipated goals differ from expected outcomes in the following ways:

1. The time span is not as long.
2. Anticipated goals are not as frequently expressed in functional terms in some facilities.
3. Anticipated goals are frequently revised.

Intervention Plan

The Intervention Plan must include the following information:

1. Frequency per day or per week that the patient will be seen (or the total number of visits that the therapist will see the patient).
2. The intervention the patient will receive.

Also frequently included are the following:

1. The location of the intervention
2. The intervention progression
3. Plans for further examination or re-examination
4. Plans for discharge
5. Plans for patient and/or family education
6. Equipment needs and equipment ordered for or sold to the patient

▌Interim/Progress Notes

Problem

The Problem section is only included in the note if there are updates or additional information regarding the medical diagnosis, test results, or medications since the most recent note was written.

Subjective (S)

Interim notes include updates or additional information regarding the patient's status since the most recent note was written.

Objective (O)

Systems Review

System Review is usually not included unless the patient's condition changes.

Reporting of Tests and Measures

Tests and Measures are updated or added to the information reported in the initial note or last interim note.

Assessment (A)

Diagnosis

Diagnosis is usually discussed in an Interim Note, or Progress Note, only if the therapy diagnosis has changed, referral to another practitioner has been made or recommended, or if the patient's functional activities or impairments change to fit a different primary or secondary practice pattern or movement dysfunction category.

Prognosis

The prognosis is usually only mentioned if the prognosis changes as a result of a change in the patient's condition.

Plan of Care (P)

Expected Outcomes

Expected Outcomes usually are not addressed in interim notes unless they have been achieved or need to be revised.

Anticipated Goals

Interim notes refer to the anticipated goals achieved and set new anticipated goals. If a goal has not yet been achieved, the notes comment on the reason the anticipated goal has not been achieved and reset the goal to make it more reasonable or restate the same goal to include a new time span.

Intervention Plan

The intervention plan needs to be revised as the patient's condition is re-examined and new anticipated goals are set.

▌Discharge Notes

Problem

The Problem section of the Discharge Notes includes updates or additional information regarding the patient's medical status, test results, or medications since the most recent note was written, *or* completely summarizes the medical history of the patient from the initial note through discharge, including test results, medications, and any other information included in this section in the initial note.

Subjective (S)

The Subjective section of the Discharge Notes includes updates or additional information regarding the patient's status since the most recent note was written, *or* completely summarizes the history of the patient from the initial note through discharge, whether the patient feels the goals set were achieved, and whether the patient feels ready to function at home or work.

Objective (O)

Systems Review

The Systems Reviews is either not mentioned at all in the Discharge Note, *or* completely summarizes the Systems Review written in the initial note.

Reporting of Tests and Measures

The Discharge Summary updates the patient's status since the last note was written, *or* completely summarizes the patient's condition upon discharge from the facility (more similar to the initial note in format and length).

Assessment (A)

Diagnosis

Diagnosis may include the following:

1. A discussion of the progression of the patient through diagnostic categories or movement dys-

function diagnoses, *or* a diagnosis section similar to the initial note
2. Referrals made to other health professionals

Prognosis

Prognosis may include the following:
1. A discussion of suggested further therapy
2. A discussion of whether or not the patient achieved the expected outcomes and anticipated goals may occur

Plan of Care (P)

Expected Outcomes

The discharge summary indicates which of the expected outcomes have been achieved and which have not been achieved (and why they were not achieved).

Anticipated Goals

In some facilities, comments are made on the most recently set anticipated goals and why they were or were not achieved. In other facilities, no comment is made on the anticipated goals.

Intervention Plan

The following information should be briefly stated:

1. Interventions delivered
2. If instruction in a home program was done and the patient's or caregiver's level of independence in the program
3. If any other type of instruction of the patient or family was performed and the level of learning that occurred (in observable terms)
4. If the patient was sold any type of equipment
5. If written instructions for any equipment sold to the patient were given
6. The number of times the patient was seen in therapy
7. Any instances of the patient skipping or canceling treatment sessions
8. If and when the patient was not seen or was put on hold and why
9. To where the patient was discharged
10. The reason from discharge from PT
11. Recommendations for follow-up interventions or care given to the patient

Tips for Note Writing for Third-Party Payers

▌ Examination

1. The current medical diagnosis and any relevant secondary medical diagnoses or test results should be included. At times, the relevant secondary medical diagnosis can help justify the need for examination of a patient's functional level, even if the patient does not need prolonged OT or PT.
2. The onset of the current medical diagnosis and the date that therapy began are essential to the D/C note.
3. *Do not* list irrelevant information. Information from the patient or significant others should help demonstrate the need for therapy.
4. When you report any complaints, keep the complaints brief and to the point. What does the patient see as his or her biggest problem? How does this problem tie into patient function (if the problem itself is not functional)?
5. Have the patient rate his or her complaints on a scale. Use of a pain scale is one example. Functional abilities at home and the amount of assistance the patient required to do them (e.g., the number of people needed) is another. Subjective information put on a type of scale can be used to re-evaluate the patient's progress.
6. Avoid listing nonspecific complaints in interim (progress) notes that are the result of normal patient discouragement. Statements like "I don't think I'm doing very well" may serve as a red flag to the reviewers and may not be validated by the results of tests and measures.
7. *Do* list the patient level of functioning prior to the onset of his or her current diagnosis. This can help justify the need for therapy in the case of a chronic illness. It can also justify the need for teaching by the therapist. (For example, a patient who has never used a walker before needs instruction in its proper use.)
8. *Do* briefly describe the patient's living environment, social history, and employment status and environment. Does the patient live alone? Who will be home during the day to care for the patient, if needed? Are there steps present, and is there a handrail? Are the steps essential for the patient to ambulate? What is the distance from the bed to the bathroom, to the kitchen, and so forth? Are the surfaces on the floors carpeted, tiled, linoleum, or hardwood, and are there any throw rugs present? Are there grab bars in the bathroom around the toilet or tub? Can a wheelchair fit through the doorways and turn in the rooms?

9. Briefly list any relevant history from the patient under the appropriate subcategories. Has the patient's functional status declined recently and why? Include whether the patient has received therapy before, why, and when. Also, has the patient ever used an assistive device before? Why and when? Does the patient own an assistive device or adaptive equipment?
10. Find out the patient's goals. What are the patient's plans upon discharge from therapy? What does he or she want to be able to do upon discharge from therapy that he or she cannot do at its initiation?
11. Measure *everything;* avoid estimates and/or terms like "appears" or "functional." All items should be quantified initially to show progress when re-examined later.
12. Show deficits that require a therapist's skilled care versus that of an aide/technician or family member. For example, show how your instruction is necessary, examine the speed of transfer and the movement of each body part during transfers, as well as the assistance needed. Only a PT or OT can work on deviations; an aide can work on mere distance and assistance.
13. Be sure to put a baseline measurement of an activity or deficit in your note if you plan an outcome or an intervention that includes that activity.
14. Show significant functional deficits and how tests and measures relate to them.
15. Be careful in reporting mental status. If you are in doubt of a patient's cognitive status, do not guess and do not emphasize the negative. A patient may be a little confused and they may be able to follow commands well and gain much benefit from therapy. Avoid terms like *confused.* If a patient is disoriented to the date, but is oriented to person, place, and task, be specific in what you state. Emphasize the patient's ability to participate in therapy.
16. Use ordinal or ratio scales (e.g., 0–10 or 0–5) to describe the results of tests and measures. It is easy for a person reading your notes to understand that 3/5 strength is deficient; "fair" strength does not imply the same level of deficiency unless the reader is trained. Include copies of rating scales used and definitions of terminology particular to your department.
17. Do not forget to take vital signs. Gait or transfer training for the sake of endurance is not reimbursable because an aide can ambulate a patient who needs only standby assistance but needs to increase ambulation distance. However, if the heart rate, blood pressure, or respiratory rate increases abnormally during

ambulation, a therapist's level of skill is needed to further train the patient in ambulation.

18. Re-examine on a regular basis. It is easier to reset goals and assess the effectiveness of interventions if consistent data are available on a regular basis.

▌Evaluation

1. Explain why a patient's progress may be slower than the usual progress made by patients with the same diagnosis.
2. Explain how impairments relate to function.

▌Plan of Care

1. Use a specific time estimate for achieving your goals. If goals are not met within an estimated time, explain why, and reset your goals.
2. Expected outcomes and anticipated goals should:
   a. Focus on *the patient* and what he or she will be able to do.
   b. State *the specific behavior* the patient will exhibit.
   c. State any *special conditions* or *equipment* needed or used: assistive devices, weight bearing status, type of wraps, prosthetics, orthotics, w/c, and so forth.
   d. Be *measurable, tied to functional activities,* and *include time frames* in which they will be achieved.
3. Be sure you continue to justify therapy as you near the completion of expected outcomes.

4. Point out progress that the patient has made toward the expected outcomes and anticipated goals as well as further goals.
5. Include the frequency with which the patient is seen.
6. Be specific enough to describe the intervention that requires a therapist versus an aide.
7. Justify the amount of time you spend with the patient by stating the type and amount of each intervention the patient receives.

▌Other

1. Make sure all forms required by the third-party payers are complete and the information required is in the appropriate section and is clear, concise, and easy to find.
2. Attach all notes required by the third-party payers. Keep yourself updated on the frequency of note writing required. Save yourself time by not writing notes any more frequently than required; progress is easier to see over a longer period.
3. For those third-party payers who required preauthorization for therapy, make sure you have preauthorization and a preauthorization number if the organization issues one. Do not exceed the number of preauthorized therapy sessions until and unless you obtain preauthorization for more therapy. Be proactive; advocate for your patient and his or her best interest with third-party payers.

Bibliography

American Physical Therapy Association: Guide to Physical Therapist Practice, ed. 2, and CD-ROM. American Physical Therapy Association, Alexandria, VA, 2002.

Baeten, AM, Moran, ML, and Phillippi, LM: Documenting Physical Therapy: The Reviewer Perspective. Butterworth-Heinemann, Boston, 1999.

Berni, R, and Ready, H: Problem-Oriented Medical Record Implementation. Allied Health Peer Review. Mosby, St. Louis, 1978.

Bernstein, F, et al: Documentation for outpatient physical therapy. Clin Man 7(2):28–30, 1987.

Common Abbreviations. Accessed at http://www.acutept.org/commonterm.html on August 13, 2003.

Feitelberg, SB: The Problem Oriented Record System in Physical Therapy. University of Vermont, Burlington, VT, 1975.

Gather, C: What your doctor doesn't know could kill you. The Boston Globe Online Magazine, 07-14-2002.

Griffith, J, and Ignatavicius, D: The Writer's Handbook: The Complete Guide to Clinical Documentation, Professional Writing and Research Papers. Resource Applications, Inc., Baltimore, 1986.

Gylys, BA, and Wedding, ME: Medical Terminology: A Systems Approach, ed. 4. F.A. Davis Company, Philadelphia, 2002.

Hill, JR: The Problem-Oriented Approach To Physical Therapy Care. American Physical Therapy Association, Washington DC, 1977.

Hughes, CJ: Tapping technology: Buying a computer. PT Magazine, June 1998, 32–36.

Hurst, JW, and Walker, HK (eds): The Problem-Oriented System. Medcom Press, 1972.

Individualized Educational Program (IEP): Individualized Educational Program: What is it/How does it work? Montgomery County Association for Retarded Citizens, Silver Springs, MD, 1978.

Instruction Objectives. Teaching Improvement Project Systems for Health Care Educators. Center for Learning Resources, College of Allied Health Professions, University of Kentucky, Lexington, KY.

Jones, P, and Oertel, W: Developing patient teaching objectives and techniques: A self-instructional program. Nurs Edu September-October, 1977, 3–18.

Kettenbach, G: Writing SOAP Notes, ed 2. F.A. Davis Company, Philadelphia, 1995.

Lew, CB: Documentation: The PT's Course on Successful Reimbursement. Professional Health Educators, Inc., Bethesda, MD, 1987.

Reynolds, JP: To compare apples with apples; Guide-based documentation. PT Magazine, June 1998, 60–71.

Rothstein, J (ed): Measurement in Physical Therapy. Churchill Livingston, Inc., New York, 1985.

Rothstein, JM, Roy, SH, and Wolf, SL: The Rehabilitation Specialist's Handbook, ed 2. F.A. Davis Company, Philadelphia, 2002.

Stewart, DL, Abeln, SH: Documenting Functional Outcomes in Physical Therapy. Mosby, St. Louis, 1993.

Wakefield, JS, and Yarnall, SR (eds): Implementing the Problem-Oriented Medical Record. MCSA, Seattle, WA, 1976.

Walter, JB, Pardee, GP, and Molbo, DM (eds): Dynamics of Problem-Oriented Approaches: Patient Care and Documentation. J.B. Lippincott Company, Philadelphia, 1976.

Weed, LL: Medical Records, Medical Education, and Patient Care. Year Book Medical Publishers, Inc., Chicago, 1971.

Weed, LL: Medical records, patient care and medical education. Ir J Med Sci 6:271–282, 1964.

Weed, LL: What physicians worry about: How to organize care of multiple problem patients. Mod Hosp 110:90–94, 1968.

Weiler, J: Documentation software: Lightening the work load. Adv Phys Ther May 18, 1998, 8–10.

Wolf, S: Clinical Decision Making in Physical Therapy. F.A. Davis Company, Philadelphia, 1985.